Transforming Lives through Women's Collectives

Role of Media in Creating Awareness on HIV/AIDS in Self-Help Groups

AF661906

Transforming Lives through Women's Collectives

Role of Media in Creating Awareness on HIV/AIDS in Self-Help Groups

Dr. S. Janet Mary

AUTHORSPRESS

Worldwide Circulation through Authorspress Global Network
First Published in 2022
by
Authorspress
Q-2A Hauz Khas Enclave, New Delhi-110 016 (India)
Phone: (0) 9818049852
E-mail: authorspressgroup@gmail.com
Website: www.authorspressbooks.com

Transforming Lives through Women's Collectives:
Role of Media in Creating Awareness on HIV/AIDS in Self-Help Groups
ISBN 978-93-5529-356-5

Copyright © 2022 Dr. S. Janet Mary

All rights reserved. No part of this book may be reproduced or transmitted in any form or by any means, electronic, mechanical, photocopying, or otherwise, without the express written consent of the author.

Printed in India at Kensington Press

Preface

Today with a billion people, India, along with Sub-Saharan Africa are the only regions in the world where over 50 percent of the deaths are still caused by infectious and wholly preventable diseases. Among the highest statistics in the world, 53 percent of the children under the age of five suffer from malnutrition, 53 percent population lives in absolute poverty, and little more than half of India's population can read.

Chennai is the capital of Tamil Nadu. It has a population of 6.6 million, of whom nearly 3 percent reside in slums located along the city's polluted waterway and railway tracks. The influence of television and cinema has been so overwhelming in Tamil Nadu that four of its Chief Ministers had their roots in the film industry. Chennai is also the headquarters of at least four Tamil satellite channels that telecast Tamil programme 24 hours a day. Given this interest in film and related media this study sees the role of media in creating HIV/AIDS awareness among the self-help group members with a particular reference to Saidapet Zone in Chennai and Keechalam in Thiruvallur Dist. HIV/AIDS prevention cannot be viewed as a onetime intervention. It must be accepted as a continuous multigenerational effort that extends well into the life time of our children and their children. The prevention or awareness programmes solely for rural areas that too among uneducated women – is lacking more in India and especially in villages of Tamil Nadu and other states. We see that they are the passive victims for no cause of their own. Another factor specially suffered by the HIV/AIDS affected uneducated women in rural areas is poverty, for their day today survival is impossible. Unlike in Africa, we see the reported cases of HIV/AIDS in rural areas in India are higher than in urban areas.

"You are not alone," self-help group members are with you" has been the core element of this thesis. Participants were interviewed regarding their demographic characteristics, sexual behaviours, and medical history.

It is my hope that this very modest work will contribute towards the reawakening of the healing power of the epidemic in the society at large.

16/2/22
(J.JANNET VENNILA)

Dr. J. JANNET VENNILA
Director - SFS (Shift II)
Madras Christian College
(Autonomous)
Tambaram, Chennai-600 059.

Acknowledgements

Words alone cannot express my appreciation for the opportunity or my indebtedness to the people whose constant guidance and assistance brought this research from an idea to a reality. But at least words can give credit where credit is due. I consider it is my pleasure to acknowledge all those individuals. First and foremost I thank the Almighty God for his goodness and blessings during the journey of my studies…

I express my deep sense of reverence and gratitude to Dr. Josephine, for her professional advice I should like to thank Dr. T. R. Gopala Krinshnan professor and head of the department, mass media and communication studies, University of Madras, Chennai who enlightened me to choose this topic and motivated me all along.

Thanks a million to my Research Guide Ms. Beuala Rachel Rajarathnamani who took a lot of personal interest to guide me all through the research. The depth of her scholarship and the richness of her intellectual insight and comments compelled me again and again to be clear in the use of concepts and more rigorous in my analysis. She helped me in myriad ways during the time of my research.

I am obliged to thank Sr. Sofi who helped me for the correct articulation of the research methodology. I express my heart felt gratitude to the respondents, who are backbone of this research for facilitating the study by co-operating and encouraging me. During the stage of writing and revising I received a lot of help and professional guidance from Mr. Amal Dass. He took special interest to read and edit the script meticulously. I should like to thank my friends who helped me to select the topic and their personnel interest shown to me.

A word of thanks weighs less but means a lot to Dr. Jennet Vennila, the Director of Madras Christian College who has written the Foreword to this volume. Finally I wish to thank all my colleagues in the Department of Communications specially Dr. Vasu, Head of the Department of Communications, Madras Christian College who has been the main brainwave for this research and publication. I take this opportunity to thank my collegues in the department of Communications in Madras Christian College who kept encouraging me all through the research.

I recall with gratitude, the dynamic vision of Ms. Dr. Bueala Racheal from Madras University, whose constant guidance and inspiration led me during the challenging journey of research.

It is my ardent duty to thank Ms.. Glenn Liza Varghese from Madras Christian College, Department of Communication who took keen interest in the final correction of this thesis.

Despite many challenges and hurdles at the end of the project I feel it is worth a go!

Dr. S. Janet Mary

Contents

CHAPTER 1

General Introduction

It is estimated that more than half of Indian population has access to the radio and television. In India Media and Communications offer a systematic introduction to any dynamic field. Starting from primary school to University level, Radio and Television play a significant role in educating and molding the children and thus the future of the country. Radio and Television have gone further in incorporating various values and morals of the society. Thus it integrates all types of people more fully into the economic, political and social mainstream of independent India. This study has attempted to bring into focus the role and significance of Radio and Television in the lives of people and how they can raise awareness in educating the rural and urban mass.

How vanquished the humankind feels in front of a virus that germinates. Acquired Immune Deficiency Syndrome AIDS is no longer a public issue but has become a serious socio-economic and developmental concern and thus there is an immediate need to act with seriousness. Each day, seven thousand young people contract HIV/AIDS. In Sahara Africa where the spread of HIV is most severe; HIV /AIDS infections are up to six times higher in young women than men of 16-24 years old. Globally there are more than 17.7 million women living with HIV, an increase of more than one million compared with two years ago. Young women are 1.6 times more likely to be living with this sickness than young men. In 2006, an estimated 39.5 million people are living with HIV and the global HIV epidemic continues to grow (*source*: The Joint United Nations Program on HIV/AIDS, World health organization). HIV affects not only the individual but also the entire generation. 4.3 million people have been infected this year alone. In the next years, it is likely to claim 120 million lives; India has second largest population of people living with HIV/AIDS, after South Africa. National AIDS Control Organization estimates that 1,24,995 Indians have HIV/AIDS. But

UNAIDS puts the figure much higher 57,00,000 Indians have HIV/AIDS. 35 percent of all reported HIV Infecs in India occur among young people between the aged of 15 and 29 (Apna Yuva Spandan National Youth Magazine Vol.1. no.1 January 2007, p. 7).

A Brief History of HIV/AIDS

On July 1981, the New York Times reported an outbreak of a rare form of cancer among gay men in New York and California, first referred to as the "gay cancer" but medically known as Kaposi sarcoma. About the same time, emergency rooms in New York City began to see a rash of seemingly healthy young men presenting with fevers, flu like symptoms, and pneumonia called pneumocystis. About a year later, the CDC (Centers for Disease Control) linked the illness to blood and coined the term as AIDS (Acquiresd Immune Deficiency Syndrome). In that first year over 1600 cases are diagnosed with close to 700 deaths.

As the number of deaths soared, medical experts scrambled to find a cause and more importantly a cure. In 1984 Pasteur institute of France discovered what they called the HIV virus, but it was not until a year later a US scientist Dr. Robert Gallo confirmed that HIV was the cause of AIDS.

Following this discovery, the first test for HIV was approved in 1985. Over the next several years medications to combat the virus were developed as well as medicines to prevent infections that flourish when the immune system is damaged by HIV and AIDS. By the end of 1987, there were 71,000 confirmed cases of AIDS resulting in over 40,000 deaths.

HIV (Human Immunodeficiency Virus) is the virus that causes AIDS:

- A – Acquired – because it's a condition one must acquire or get infected with, not something transmitted through the genes.
- I – Immune – because it affects the body's immune system, the part of the body which usually works to fight off germs such as bacteria and viruses.
- D – Deficiency – because it makes the immune system deficient (makes it not work properly)

- S – Syndrome – because someone with AIDS may experience a wide range of different diseases and opportunitistic infections from one person to another through blood-to-blood and sexual contact. In addition infected pregnant woman can pass HIV to their baby during pregnancy or delivery, as well as through breast-feeding. People with HIV have what is called HIV infection. Many of these people will develop AIDS as a result of their HIV infection.

Infectious "bodily fluids" proven to spread HIV:

- blood
- semen
- vaginal fluid
- breast milk
- other body fluids containing blood
- "bodily fluids" Non-infectious:
    - saliva
    - tears
    - sweat
    - faces
    - urine

The first case of HIV/AIDS was reported in Tamil Nadu, India in 1986. Since then the virus has spread from the high-risk groups to the general population very fast. Today there are 5.7 million people living with HIV/AIDS in India.

Women and children are increasingly becoming vulnerable to HIV/AIDS. The new findings conclude that 38% of the infected people shifted from 55 (per 100 males) in 2001 to 60 in 2005. This indicated the increasing feminization of HIV/AIDS in India.

This alarming trend is being observed closely as more HIV positive mothers will unknowingly pass the virus on to their children. The incidence of parent to child transmission jumped from 2.7% to 3.5% in just one year. The current HIV/AIDS programme are reaching only 15% of young people and 17% of high risk group sub-population such as sex workers, men who have sex with men and injecting drug users.

Women and HIV/AIDS in India

Most issues that affect positive women are similar to that of men living with HIV but the impact may be different. Women are more vulnerable to HIV infection because of several factors including social, gender, and economic and biological ones. Patriarchal society, economic dependency and gender imbalance are the main reasons for the increased vulnerability of women HIV/AIDS is fuelled by discrimination and repression in many ways.

The women sex workers are more vulnerable because of poverty, the economic disparity, stigma attached to their profession, lack of skills to make a living and lack of knowledge to stand for their rights. Young women who had supported themselves as sex workers wasted away from AIDS related infections. The woman literacy in our country is low and they never get to know of HIV/AIDS and their own HIV status till they reach chronic and acute stage.

Women face more rejection by the family than men; they are the most disadvantaged members of the family. Some people consider that only those who have multiple partners are at risk. It is true that the risk increases with. Even when wives are aware that their husbands had contracted AIDS through extra marital relationship they continue to care for them. As the psychological effects of being infected with HIV, the women fall into depression, anxiety and many are led to suicidal tendency.

Background and Context

Today with a billion people, India, along with Sub-Saharan Africa are the only regions in the world where over 50 percent of the deaths are still caused by infectious and wholly preventable diseases. Among the highest statistics in the world, 53 percent of the children under the age of five suffer from malnutrition, 53 percent population lives in absolute poverty, and little more than half of India's population can read.

Chennai is the capital of Tamil Nadu. It has a population of 6.6 million, of whom nearly 3 percent reside in slums located along the city's polluted waterway and railway tracks. The influence of television and cinema has been so overwhelming in Tamil Nadu that four of its Chief Ministers had their roots in the film industry. Chennai is also the headquarters of at least four Tamil satellite channels that telecast Tamil programme 24 hours a day. Given this interest in film and related media this study will see the role of media in creating HIV/AIDS awareness among the self-help group members with a particular reference to Saidapet Zone in Chennai and Keechalam in Thiruvallur Dist. HIV/AIDS prevention cannot be viewed as a onetime intervention. It must be accepted as a continuous multigenerational effort that extends well into the life time of our children and their children. The prevention or awareness programmes solely for rural areas that too among uneducated women – is lacking more in India and especially in villages of Tamil Nadu and other states. We see that they are the passive victims for no cause of their own. Another factor specially suffered by the HIV/AIDS affected uneducated women in rural areas is poverty, for their day today survival is impossible. Unlike in Africa, we see the reported cases of HIV/AIDS in rural areas in India are higher than in urban areas.

Self-Help Group

Self-Help is a way to deal with problems that everyone faces from time to time in their lives illness, divorce, and the death of a loved one, emotional upsets or strains. Talking over these problems with other people who have lived through them can help us cope with today's difficulties and help us learn how to deal with tomorrow.

Helping is at the centre of all this activity: knowing how to receive help give help and help yourself. Underlying self-help is the basic theme. "You are not alone," self-help group members are with you.

- Feel less isolated knowing others share similar problems:
- Exchange ideas and effective ways to cope with problems:
- Actively work in their attitudes and behavior to make positive changes in their lives.
- Gain a new sense of control over their lives.

The knowledge base of self-help mutual support groups is experiential, indigenous and rooted in the wisdom that comes from struggling with problems in concrete, shared ways. Self – help groups build on the strengths of their members.

In Tamil Nadu Context

SHG is group of rural poor who have volunteered to organize themselves into a group for eradication of poverty of the members.

They agree to save regularly and convert their savings into a Common Fund known as the Group corpus. The members of the group agree to use this common fund and such other funds that they may receive as a group through a common management. The group formation will keep in view the following broad guidelines:

Generally a self-help group may consist of 10 to 20 persons. However, in difficult areas like deserts, hills and areas with scattered and sparse population and in case of minor irrigation and disabled persons, this number may be from 5-20. The difficult areas have to be identified by the State Level SGSY Committee and the above relaxation in membership will be permitted only in such areas.

Generally all members of the group should belong to families below the poverty line. However, if necessary, a maximum of 20% and in exceptional cases, where essentially required, up to a maximum of 30% of the members in a group may be taken from families marginally above the poverty line living contiguously with BPL families and if they are acceptable to the BPL members of the group. This will help the families of occupational groups like agricultural labourers, marginal farmers and artisans marginally above the poverty line, or who may have been excluded from the BPL list to become members of the Self Help Group. However, the APL members will not be eligible for the subsidy under the scheme. The group shall not consist of more than one member from the same family. A person should not be a member of more than one group. The BPL families must actively participate in the management and decision making, which should not ordinarily be entirely in the hands of APL families. Further, APL members of the Self Help Group shall not become office bearers (Group Leader, Assistant Group Leader or Treasurer) of the Group.

The group should devise a code of conduct (Group management norms) to bind itself. This should be in the form of regular meetings (weekly or fortnightly), functioning in a democratic manner, allowing free exchange of views, participation by the members in the decision making process.

The group should be able to draw up an agenda for each meeting and take up discussions as per the agenda.

The members should build their corpus through regular savings. The group should be able to collect the minimum voluntary saving amount from all the members regularly in the group meetings. The savings so collected will be the group corpus fund.

The group corpus fund should be used to advance loans to the members. The group should develop financial management norms covering the loan sanction procedure, repayment schedule and interest rates.

The members in the group meetings should take all the loaning decisions through a participatory decision making process.

The group should be able to priorities the loan applications, fix repayment schedules, fix appropriate rate of interest for the loans advanced and closely monitor the repayment of the loan installments from the loanee.

The group should operate a group account preferably in their service area bank branch, so as to deposit the balance amounts left with the groups after disbursing loans to its members.

The group should maintain simple basic records such as Minutes book, Attendance register, Loan ledger, General ledger, Cash book, Bank passbook and individual passbooks. The sample preformed for maintenance of above records by the group is in the Annexure II for guidance. These could be used with necessary changes/ modifications wherever required.

50% of the groups formed in each block should be exclusively for the women. In the case of disabled persons, the groups formed should ideally be disability-specific wherever possible, however, in case sufficient number of people for formation of disability-specific groups are not available, a group may comprise of persons with diverse disabilities or a group may comprise of both disabled and non-disabled persons below the poverty line.

As Tiruvallur district is predominantly agricultural district, construction of threshing floors will go a long way in helping the farming community.

How SHG Can Help In AIDS

The members of the self-help group have been trained by the DMI (NGO). Since they have been trained in the methods of prevention of this disease and also the curative aspect, they can easily contact the local people and explain the preventive and the curative aspects of this disease. Social awareness can be created by SHG because they know the tactics to deliver proper information to the people. Since they meet the local people often the contact can be permanent. Added to the media information the SHG's can easily impart important information to the local people.

Conceptualization

The study of awareness of the seriousness of HIV/AIDS among SHG could be conceptualized in concepts such as:

- HIV/AIDS patients
- Self-help group in rural and urban
- Role of media to bring awareness

The Role of Media in HIV/AIDS Awareness Creation in Tamil Nadu

While addressing the media leaders' summit on HIV/AIDS, the Prime Minister

Dr. Man Mohan Singh stressed on strengthening the national AIDS control as commitment of the national common minimum programme. He emphasized the need for supplementing all such efforts with an active and avid participation from all sections of the society culmination in a mass movement for creating awareness of HIV/AIDS.

In June 2001, at UN General Assembly Special Session on HIV/AIDS, as landmark gathering, the Heads of the state and representatives of Governments affirmed that:

> Beyond the key role played by communities, strong partnerships among governments, the United Nations system... People living with AIDS and vulnerable groups… the media, parliamentarians, foundations community organizations and traditional leaders are important.

The media has the potential to create widespread awareness on HIV/AIDS to promote the positive attitude towards people living with HIV/AIDS and also influencing people to change high risk behavior that make them vulnerable infection.

According to a survey conducted in India, 70% of Indians identified television a primary source of information about HIV/AIDS. At the United Nations assembly special session on HIV/AIDS in June 2001 it was agreed by the government of the state that:

> By 2005 ensure that 90% and by 2010, 95% of youth aged 15-24 have information, education, services and life skills that enable them to reduce their vulnerability to HIV.

Hence, an effective media can raise the awareness level and can also bring about sustainable behavior change there by reducing vulnerability to the virus. The media has the potential to influence public opinion and attitudes about HIV/AIDS. Media too have the capability to bring transformation in the thinking pattern of the society in sowing the seeds of attitudinal changes. The media can be a great facilitator for preventing awareness in the society.

Information is power and that awareness that empowers. According to UNAIDS and the world health organization, as many as two of new HIV infective projected to occur globally by 2010 could be averted more effective prevention and public education efforts. The practical and fast way in which one can change anything is through media. India has the large and powerful media group which pledged its participation in the nation for HIV awareness campaign.

Effective media coverage personalizes the HIV issue, encourages people to interact and share their views, which in turn prompts the government to prioritize the HIV/AIDS issue in the social and political agenda. An effective coverage enforces the element of accountability and a sense of responsibility to encourage the people to raise their voices.

Media combats the disease through public education and awareness as the disease is not only a battle against a virus but is also a battle against the social discrimination, cultural taboo and the ideas.

Media is contributing in a global fight against HIV/AIDS as it plays an essential role in reversing the progression of HIV/AIDS. Though media has enormous potential to undertake the challenge of fighting with AIDS but to perform its responsibility with utmost efficiency requires the clear understanding of the challenge and the obstacles to spread the education about AIDS. The media have an important role to play in raising awareness in combating "compassion fatigue" and focusing attention or what is being done and what more must be done. It is no longer someone else's problem. It is life a death challenge of our times and we are all affected even if we are all infected.

The status of women in India can only be improved through a join – programme between the media and the community in providing Indian women with the power of literacy. Women in India are divided into unequal halves. Of 368 million women in India, 278 reside in rural areas and most are illiterate. The majority of illiterate women number 75%, 25% is semi – literate, and 5% may be considered educated. In an effort to integrate women into the mainstream of Indian social life a campaign of providing literacy to all women has been undertaken. It has gone further in incorporating the media in educating people regarding these various social ills and evils of the society.

Scope of Study

Today the media is under used regarding the awareness programmes for anyone especially women. They cash on their usual sentiments and emotions and produce serials and mega-serials which really kill their time. It diverts them from many more serious issues in the society, especially for women. Many women themselves are not convinced of the need of a celebration of the international women's day though the women make up about 50% of humanity, they own only 1% of the properties in the world. A number of serious issues about violence against women at homes, working places denial of their salaries, sex trafficking and issues on Dalit women and so on.

Since media in Tamil Nadu especially the political parties have made it clear to distribute to all homes, also the daily newspapers with the periodical magazines mushrooming in the readers market, have made the media and communications cheaper than a cup of tea. Many ways the media has made powerful in road into the daily lives of people. The 24 hours networking of television programmes has taken over the lives and culture of the people. This has to be effectively used to propagate lots of awareness to the people. As for as the AIDS is concerned a lot of misunderstanding is passed around. The issues on AIDS must be given a very creative and innovative way through the media so that they show interest to see them in the television or read in the newspapers.

The studies of awareness of the disease among women are limited and date available is not country specific because of the varying differences in economic, sociological, medical and public health conditions. Therefore, this particular approach needs to be critically evaluated, of the role of media in spreading awareness among women in general and women in Tamil Nadu in particular for the state is booming with the patients of this deadly virus day by day. Women need to be educated and made aware of the ways and means of contracting this disease and the ways and means to overcome it. A good number of women are aware that the main way to contract the transmit of this disease is through sexual intercourse but there other misunderstandings regarding pregnancy, menstrual behavior, breastfeeding etc. which are to be made known to them through various means of mass media and communications.

Objectives of the Study

General Objectives

- To find out the respondents, awareness on role of media in creating awareness about the cause and consequences of HIV/AIDS.

Specific Objectives

- To find out respondents awareness on preventive measures against HIV/AIDS through media.
- To find out the sources of information on HIV/ AIDS among SHG due to media dissemination.
- To analyze the positive attitude towards AIDS affected people due to media influences.

Hypothesis

- Media has the potential to create widespread awareness on HIV/AIDS to promote the positive attitude among self-help groups.
- Higher the education of respondent greater the level of awareness through media.
- The preventive measures of HIV/AIDS are the role of media influence.
- Positive attitude towards AIDS affected people is due to media dissemination.

CHAPTER 2

Review of Literature

The whole world has understood the seriousness of the killer disease HIV/AIDS. Hence the governments of all the countries are seized of this problem and are taking steps to prevent the spread of the same. But the NGO's play a major role in educating the people aided by the media. Hence it was planned to undertake study on the role of media in creating awareness on HIV/AIDS among the people. Even in this it was decided to study the part played by the women especially the SHG members in Tamil Nadu.

Though these SHG groups were formed among the women for the economic uplift of the women folk, considering the seriousness of HIV/AIDS the NGO's and the government wished that they also should take part in this uphill tasks of creating awareness among the people about the harmful effects of this disease. There is considerable amount of success too.

"When you are working to combat disastrous and growing emergency, you should use every tool at your disposal. HIV/AIDS is the worst epidemic humankind ever faced. It has spread further faster and with more catastrophic longer term effects than any other disease. It is impact has become a devastating obstacle to development. Broadcast media have tremendous reach and influence, particularly with young people who represent the future and who hold the key to much successful fight against HIV/AIDS. We must seek to engage in powerful originations as full partners in the fight to halt HIV/AIDS through awareness, prevention and education. "*Kofi Annan, United Nations Former Secretary General*".

> *The article HIV/AIDS prevention and creating awareness and the role of media* gives us vivid facts about the role of media that has to be played in creating awareness among the people.

An article entitled "An innovative approach to reducing HIV/AIDS prevalence through targeted mass media communications in Mumbai, India", focuses on need for dissemination of related information and realities pertaining to the epidemic so that the ignorance is replaced by awareness and then creating multiplied effects of awareness engulfing the wider cross sections of the society. The article states that India poised on the precipice of devastating HIV/AIDS epidemic. Twenty years after the first case of AIDS was reported in India now come to second largest number of HIV infected people in the world around 51 million people as in 2003 being infected by the deadly disease. Despite ardent efforts to proliferate awareness of HIV/AIDS being made by governmental and non-governmental agencies, the misconceptions relating HIV/AIDS continue to outpace the efforts to educate people regarding the disease. Thus, with the passage of time role of media has become increasingly significant.

Task before visual and non-visual vehicles of media besides creating awareness and providing knowledge base about HIV/AIDS is also to remove the misconceptions about the transmission of the virus and the social ostracisms affected persons.

Countries such as Thailand that have recorded declining trends of HIV/AIDS infection have demonstrated that this pandemic beats a retreat in the face determined and sustained massive efforts in generating awareness among people, and empowering people with information to combat it effectively.

The media has the potential to create widespread awareness on HIV/AIDS to promote the positive attitudes towards people living with HIV/AIDS.

Here it will be or appropriate to quote the speech delivered by Dr. Man Mohan Sing, our Prime Minister at the Media Leaders' summit on HIV/AIDS on 6th January 2005:

> "From one reported HIV case in 1986, the number of HIV positive people in India has already crossed the five million mark. HIV/AIDS is no longer just a public health issue, as my colleague the Health Minister mentioned just a moment ago, it has become a serious socio-economic and developmental concern. If not checked, it can hurt our ambitions in economic growth and development very severely. Though HIV/AIDS can affect everyone, it is often the poor, youth and women in distress who are most vulnerable. We have no choice but to act, and act with firmness, with urgency and with utmost seriousness.

While focusing attention on research for finding a vaccine for this pandemic, we must leave no stone unturned in preventing its occurrence by using media in an intelligent and creative manner. In the absence of a vaccine, the social vaccine of education and awareness is the only preventive tool we have. It is appropriately said that prevention begins with information. Media, which conveys information and moulds public opinion, must remain at the heart of our campaign to help people make informed choices.

Visibility in the media, and informed and sympathetic visibility at that, is a first step towards creating greater awareness. Leaders of media, in alliance with other segments of our polity and society, can play a significant role in educating public opinion. All of you are aware that there are many misconceptions about AIDS that need to be dispelled. Half information is often more dangerous than no information.

I would like to urge you to transmit your messages in all Indian languages so that they reach the widest cross section of our society. While as a public service broadcaster, Doordarshan has a special role to play, I do believe that all media should be pro-active. I am encouraged by the presence here of many important private sector media organizations. I commend you for your interest and commitment".

Many scholars have studied this aspect of spreading awareness and their findings have helped in evolving conclusions about this subject. "VISION U.S. agency initiated a Project which aimed to increase use of family survival and HIV/AIDS services. The VISION project used a mass media campaign of reproductive health and HIV/AIDS prevention. They conducted detailed analysis based on a data from 2002-2004 collected in Nigeria.

The results of findings were Socio-demographic characteristics of the population are presented in Table 1. The average age (28.1) of the respondents and the mean number of sexual partners in the past year (1.2) were similar across states. In Bauchi, 73% of the respondents were married; 45% reported being married in Enugu and 60% reported being married in Oyo. Seventy-four percent of respondents in Oyo reported living in urban or peri-urban areas; 35% of respondents in Bauchi and 36% of respondents in Enugu reported living in urban or peri-urban areas. The states also differed in educational attainment, with Bauchi reporting the lowest proportion of respondents reporting secondary or higher education (20.4%) and Enugu reporting the highest proportion of respondents reporting secondary or higher education (60%). Oyo had the highest proportion of Protestants/other Christians (55%), Bauchi had the highest number of Muslims (89%), and Enugu had the highest proportion of Catholics (71%). Knowledge of a condom source also varied by state, with 57% of respondents in Oyo, and 51% and 26% of respondents in Enugu and Bauchi, respectively, reporting that they know where to get condoms.(Enugu, Oyo and Bauchi are selected places in Nigeria.)

The conclusion arrived at was, the data shows that the FP/RH media campaign by VISION and its partners is reaching a large portion of the target population, and exposure to these mass media programs can help increase HIV/AIDS awareness. Programs that target rural populations, females, and unmarried individuals, as well as disseminate information on where to obtain condoms, are needed to reduce barriers to condom use. Although the overall differences in the outcome variables between 2002 baseline data and 2004 follow-up data were small, differences in the outcome variables observed in the respective project areas for sub-groups of the population suggest that change is starting to occur. Improvements in HIV/AIDS prevention behaviour are likely to require that these programmatic efforts be continued, scaled up, done in conjunction with other interventions, and targeted towards individuals or areas with specific socio-demographic characteristics.

A Research Study undertaken by the Tamil Nadu AIDS control Society Clearly shows the Importance of Awareness Programmes

Awareness is the key to the prevention and control of HIV / AIDS. Fear is not likely to solve any of the problems, neither is ignorance. The electronic, print and other media are fully exploited, optimizing the use of the resources of TANSACS. The first phase of the IEC campaign has been a resounding success, as independent surveys of professional agencies have indicated. The campaign is already being hailed as a model for the other states in the subcontinent. The emphasis has shifted towards interpersonal communication and behaviour change communication to ensure positive behavioural changes.

Many Non-Governmental organizations (NGOs) are involved in creating awareness, and implementing intervention programmes. TANSACS has identified several demographic groups with risk-prone lifestyles such as CSWs, truckers and migrant workers. It has initiated several targeted intervention projects through the NGOs to promote safe sex behaviour and condom use among groups with high-risk behaviour. 98 intervention projects were implemented so far in the state in urban and rural areas.

The Impact Created by these Interactions by the Social Workers is Very Important in creating awareness

The data on knowledge indicators was analysed separately for those who had an interaction with social workers (such as Health Workers, Counsellors, NGOs etc.) and those who did not have an interaction with social workers.

From this table, it is clearly evident that the knowledge levels are significantly higher among the respondents who received information from the social worker / counsellor on a one to one basis. On the whole, it can be concluded that increased focus on mass media may not necessarily lead to a considerable change in the knowledge and behaviour of the population sub-groups. However, personal one to one interaction with specific groups like Social workers, Counsellors, Doctors and NGOs might be more effective in dealing with the misconceptions of people and in educating them, particularly with regard to the spread and prevention of HIV/ AIDS.

Summary

Television is the most preferred media, followed by Radio.

Awareness on HIV/AIDS is higher than the awareness on STD/RTI.

Major source of information on HIV/AIDS was through TV, Radio.

A Research Paper on Role of media on HIV awareness in Tamil Nadu Stated when Mentioning about the Role of Communication in HIV Prevention States

"The most effective prevention messages or which help provide skills to be used interpersonally regarding refusal, delay, and negotiation are ability to say no when pressured to have sex, to put off sex if unwanted, and to negotiate to use condoms. Role plays, rehearsals, etceteraed, are most critical. Unfortunately, politics, religion, are supposed values often get in the way of delivering the messages that would be most likely to succeed: 'remain abstinent if you can, but learn how to negotiate for condom use if you're already active."'

This research covered wide areas both rural and urban and a number of different categories of people like.

Sample size Population of Sub-Groups

Commercial sex workers (CSW), Migrant labourers, Truck drivers, Students, Men having sex with men(MSM), Prisoners, Street children, IV Drug Users

Different Kinds of Media were Studied for this Purpose

The main media from where HIV/ AIDS messages are recalled: Health workers NGOs, TV, Radio Stickers behind buses and autos, direct contact with health workers, Hoarding, wall painting, written material like pamphlets, hand-outs, Play, Drama.

In general, the awareness levels on STD/ HIV/ AIDS are considerably high among all the population sub-groups surveyed. Obviously, the high awareness levels can be attributed to the interventions done through mass media like TV, radio, cinema and newspaper/ magazine in the past few years. It is a well-known fact that mass media vehicles are very effective in creating general awareness levels of the disease (viz. spreading horizontal knowledge). However, these mass media vehicles have limited application in imparting in-depth vertical knowledge. Interestingly, the data clearly shows that personal attention actually increases the depth of knowledge related to the spread and prevention of HIV/ AIDS, which is very important

The data on knowledge indicators was analyzed separately for those who had an interaction with social workers (such as Health Workers, Counsellors, NGOs etc.) and those who did not have an interaction with social workers. From this table, it is clearly evident that the knowledge levels are significantly higher among the respondents who received information from the social worker / counsellor on an one to one basis. On the whole, it can be concluded that increased focus on mass media may not necessarily lead to a considerable change in the knowledge and behaviour of the population sub-groups. However, personal one to one interaction with specific groups like Social workers, Counsellors, Doctors and NGOs might be more effective in dealing with the misconceptions of people and in educating them, particularly with regard to the spread and prevention of HIV/ AIDS.

Television is the most preferred media, followed by Radio. Awareness on HIV/AIDS is higher than the awareness on STD/RTI. Major source of information on HIV/AIDS was through TV, radio, panels and newspapers.

Awareness level varies from group to group, not uniform. Knowledge levels are higher in the high risk behavior groups than the low risk population.

Knowledge levels are high in individuals who are interacted with social workers. Majority feels that the government should provide HIV/AIDS related education on a constant basis.

"Nalamdana" (Are you well?) is an organization started in 1993 by people belong to various profession to teach healthy life to people through methods like street theatre, discussion groups and songs with messages.

The group is involved in

- Researching, scripting and performing community drama to increase awareness of key health and social issues and positive behaviour change; Development of television dramas on social issues;
- Development of Information, Education and Communication (IEC) materials for awareness and behavior change;
- Conducting workshops on awareness about STDs and HIV, especially for illiterate men and women;
- Facilitating fund raising for and the dissemination of *Nalamdana* Scholarship Funds;
- Building up resources by training college students in street theatre.

They are Confident that Significant Changes can be Effected by the Atrical Means

An evaluation of *Nalamdana* the artical activities showed that a significant increase in HIV/AIDS-related knowledge occurred as a result of watching the drama. Before the play, audiences had relatively high levels of accurate knowledge about HIV/AIDS, but lower knowledge levels of common HIV/AIDS misconceptions. The drama reduced these misconceptions and also increased the level of reported intentions to treat HIV – positive individuals more kindly.

Considerable misinformation existed with regard to HIV/AIDS knowledge. The pre-test sensitization analysis showed that the pre-test may have accounted for not more than four percent of this inaccurate knowledge increase. Importantly, there were differences in baseline HIV/AIDS knowledge such that certain low-income areas had lower levels of HIV/AIDS knowledge. These lower knowledge areas had greater increased in knowledge and thus the drama served to reduce this knowledge gap. The knowledge gap that exists between lower and higher SES groups can thus be reduced with interventions, such as community-level drama that appeals to the audience and communicates information in a manner that is understandable

From all these research papers and other investigative reports it is understood that the media can play a major role in disseminating information about this killer disease. But one thing is absent here and that is the personal touch. If a person with some knowledge in the subject is met face, to face one can raise questions and immediately get the answer. That is why SHG members were identified to gain knowledge about the awareness that had spread among the people about this disease. This can be ever quoted as one of the successful studies conducted on this subject.

Social Learning Theory (Albert Bandura)

Social learning theory is a general theory of human behavior, but Bandura and people concerned with mass communication have used it specially to explain media effects. Bandura warned that "children and adults acquire attitudes, emotional responses, and new styles of conduct through filmed and televised modeling. Bandura says it is fortunate that people learn from vicarious observation, since mistakes could prove costly or fatal. This theory is implied in my research as how the media has created an impact in the minds of people or how it has created an impression in the mind of the people that HIV/AIDS is a serious disease.

CHAPTER 3

Methodology

The validity of a research study to a great extent lies in the methodology. An enquiry would be neither valid nor reliable if it is not done along certain methodological line. Research methodology is a way to solve the research problem systematically. It may be understood as a science of studying how research is done scientifically. In it we study the various steps that are generally made by a researcher in studying the research problem along with the logic behind them. This is necessary for the researcher to know not only the research method techniques, but also the methodology. Social research has developed as a body of scientific principles and techniques, which are being applied recent origin and applied more and more to the study and an analysis of social problems constitute a part of research methodology. So the researcher has used the following methods in order to study the research problem.

The Study

The study was conducted in a systematic manner so as to find out the level of awareness fashioned by media on HIV/AIDS among the Self-Help Group of rural and urban set up.

Research Design

A research design is the logical and systematic plan prepared for directing a research study. It is the arrangement of conditions for collection and analysis of data in a manner that aims to combine relevance to the research purpose with economy in procedures.

In fact the conceptual structure within which the research is conducted and it constitutes the blue print for the collection, measurement and analysis of data. As such the research design includes the details about the problem, the objectives, and research questions of the study, sampling plan and method and techniques of data collection. Thus the research design spells out in considerable detail what occur in the following steps of the research.

This research is based on data from the self-help groups of Saidapet area of Chennai and Keechalam in Chengelpet Dist as rural area. The study was conducted among 300 respondents between the age group of 25-45. To be more scientific and accurate along with the questionnaire a descriptive method was also followed on HIV/AIDS. This study describes the level of knowledge of respondents in relation to the causes, symptoms and prevention of HIV. The media has the potential to create widespread awareness on HIV/AIDS to promote the positive attitudes towards people living with AIDS. It has a pivotal role to play in a fight against AIDS. Education is the vaccine against AIDS. With the passage of time role of media has become increasingly significant in Tamil Nadu. Hence the people of Saidapet zone in Chennai Keechalam in Chengelpet area will be a descriptive study based on the response received from the scientific questionnaire.

Descriptive Research Design

Research designs are closely linked with the objectives of a research problem. So the research design of the present study is a descriptive research design.

Descriptive study is a fact-finding investigation with adequate interpretation. It describes as accurately as possible the characteristic of a group of people or a community. It is designed to gather descriptive information and provides information for formulating sophisticated studies.

Methods of Data Collection

Primary and secondary data were collected for this study. The primary data was collected from 300 respondents, through a self-structured survey questioner. The secondary data was collected from books, periodicals, magazines and internet for the study.

Tools of Data Collection

The tool for data collection is a probability sampling method close ended questions. The data collection was divided into two parts; the first part consists of the profile of the respondents describing their socio-economic background and the second part consists of questions regarding the role of media creating awareness on the seriousness of HIV/AIDS. Each question has fixed / limited with choices. Participants, observation style were also followed.

Sampling Method

Single unit of study is referred to as an element of population. When we select a group of elements for the purpose of study of a particular phenomenon, we refer to that group of elements for the purpose of study of a particular phenomenon; we refer to that group of elements as a sample. The results obtained from the sample are more precise and correct than the results obtained from the study of the whole group. Sometimes it is not feasible to study a whole group or an extremely large group. The sample study of a large population can, in practice produce more valid and reliable than can a censes.

The study has been undertaken in the urban and rural set up of Chennai and Thiruvallur districts respectively. The researcher followed simple questionnaire sampling method for collecting data from 150 respondents respectively. With the consent of the Chairperson of Daughters of Mary Immaculate (DMI) the NGO that is operative in these two areas, the data was collected in Keechalam and Saidapet.

Keechalam

Keechalam is a vibrant village near Thiruthani under Thiruvallur District of Tamil Nadu. It is 105 kilo meters away from the capital city of Chennai. Geographically this area is located near the border of Andhra Pradesh. Obviously the people speak both Tamil and Telugu. There are four blocks in this district of which for the research, Pallipet Taluk have been selected for the survey. They are mostly agriculturists, however many also involve in candle making, tailoring, weaving and leather works. Daughters of Mary Immaculate (DMI) an international NGO by women religious group has been working in this area for the past 20 years. The target group has been women to empower and animate them. Amazingly DMI has spread its wings in 10 districts of Tamil Nadu with its overwhelming activities of empowerment and awareness programmes. This NGO has formed 555 women groups only in this area. I have chosen only 22 groups for my sample study. Though each group has its own name, generally they are called Mahalir Kuzhu. Each group has 12-20 members.

AREA OF STUDY

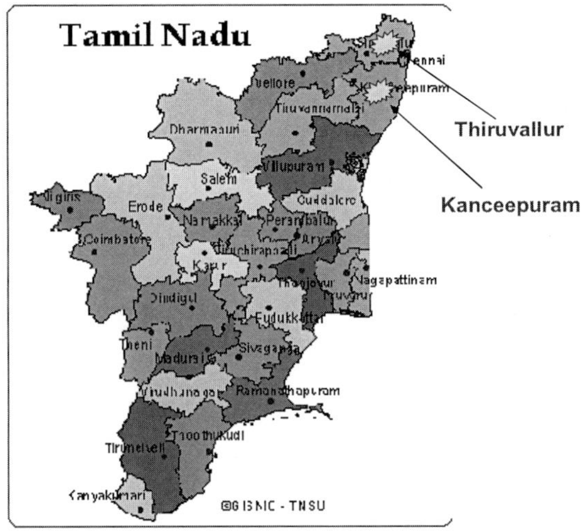

Saidapet

Saidapet is one of the southern suburban regions of Chennai city. The place is situated off the Anna Salai Road in the southern precincts of the city. MGR Nager, Adyar and Kotturpuram are the neighbouring city outskirts. Saidapet is basically a residential area and with provisions are requisite to meet the demands of the local population. The place is about 8kms from the Chennai Central Railway Station and lies in the referral point. The Daughters of Mary Immaculate (DMI) an international NGO by women religious group has been working in this area for the past one year. They have formed 20 women self-help groups. These women along with their families have been migrated from the southern states of Tamil Nadu such as, Kanya Kumari, Thirunelvelli, and Madurai. Their main entertainment is watching Television most of the time. Some eight groups have taken loans through Mahalir Kuzhu and have started minor scale businesses.

The Purpose of SHG

The arms of the Government cannot reach each and every corner of the country. Hence the Government had thought about forming Self Help Groups almost in all villages. Though these groups were formed to improve the economic status of women, gradually they started dealing with the social aspects of the village. Any progress in society will not be possible if women are not involved in the activities. Nowaday's women play a significant role in the society as teachers and educators. When they form a group it becomes more effective.

Coming to the point of AIDS, to some extent women are the worst affected section of the society. Hence it is better they are educated by women. Since certain aspects of this disease are a little delicate to discuss openly, women are the better people to spread the information regarding this disease. This is still easily done by groups. Self-help groups can do the work easily because they know the economic and social conditions of the locals and their education background also. They can select suitable methods for each set of people to get the information.

Last but not the least; the SHGs are wielding considerable importance in the locality. Hence I very strongly feel that they are the fittest people to spread this awareness about AIDS.

Types of Sampling Method

The research followed the probability sampling method to find out the profile of the respondents and to measure the level of media awareness of respondents on the effect of HIV/AIDS. Probability sampling specifies the chances that the sample statistics do not differ more than a certain limit from the population parameters.

Data Analysis and Processing

The collected data was coded in to numbers and entered into a master sheet. Then based on the researcher's hypothesis, tables were made and statistical tests were carried out and analyzed.

CHAPTER 4

Analysis and Interpretation

Introduction

The researcher has examined the Role of Media in creating awareness on HIV/AIDS among the rural areas of Keechalam and the urban area of Saidapet, with the Self Help Groups. The researcher has pin-pointed the areas on age, education, occupation and income variable scales. The responses derived from the data were listed in tables unique to every question. All the responses were recorded in the tables in different level scales. These tables were categorized accordingly to the working hypothesis. For each hypothesis, responses of the questions were tabulated to determine the average in order to test the hypothesis formulated.

Social Background of The Study

A study of general background of 150 women respondents is presented in this research. It will enable us to understand clearly the diverse factors affecting the value orientation of the respondents and the general background of the respondents in an important variable in the research.

I. Age

Age is chronological which shows the length of life on existence. It reflects wisdom and maturity. Age can be defined as the attainment of mental status and knowledge attained by an individual.. Age plays an important role for the growth and experience through which knowledge is acquired. Thus AGE is taken into the study in order to see whether there is association or relationship between age and awareness in relation to media on HIV/AIDS.

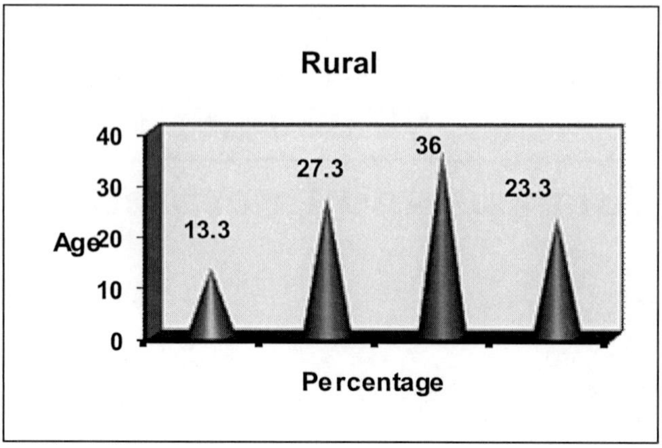

Age Rural

DESCRIPTION	RESPONDENT	PERCENTAGE
20-25	20	13.3
25-30	41	27.3
30-35	54	36.0
35 and above	35	23.3
TOTAL	**150**	**100.0**

The Self Help age group is from 20 to 35 and above. Table – 1, we come to know that 13.3 percent of respondents were in the age group of 20 to 25. Then 27.3 percent of respondents were in the age group of 25 to 30 years. 36 percent of respondents were in the age group of 30 to 35 years. 23.3 percent of them were between the age group of 35 and above.

The maximum of 36 per cent of respondents were in the category of age group between 30 to 35 years and the lower age group (20 to 25) is only 13.3 per cent. It is interesting to note that most (36%) of them are rather middle-aged persons. Hence the exposure to media and its awareness must be better among this group than the lower age group.

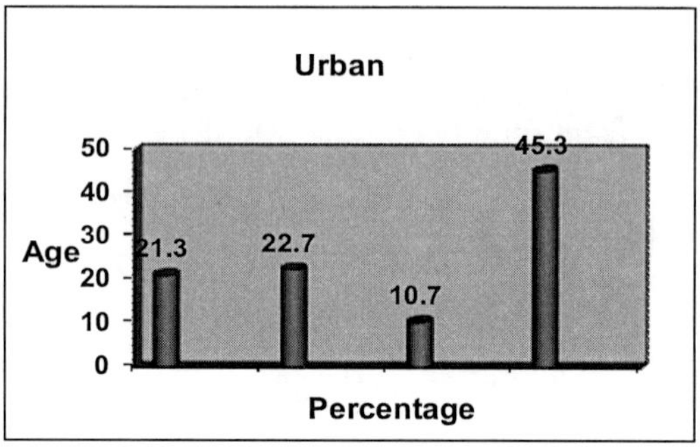

Description	Respondent	Percentage
20-25	32	21.3
25-30	34	22.7
30-35	16	10.7
Above 35	68	45.3
Total	**150**	**100**

The Self Help age group is from 20 to 35 and above. Table – 1, we come to know that 21.3 percent of respondents were in the age group of 20 to 25. Then 22.7 percent of respondents were in the age group of 25 to 30 years. 10.7 percent of respondents were in the age group of 30 to 35 years. 45.3 percent of them were between the age group of 35 and above.

The maximum of 45.3 percent of respondents were in the category of age group between above 35 years and the lower age group (30 to 35) is only 10.7 percent. It is interesting to note that most (45.3%) of them are rather middle-aged persons. Hence the exposure to media and its awareness must be better among this group than the lower age group.

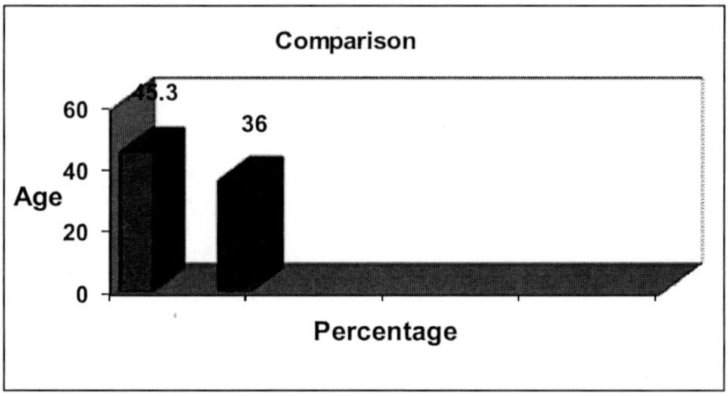

In urban areas 45.3% of the persons of the age group between 30 to 35 are better aware of this HIV/AIDS than the other age groups. In rural areas nearly 36% of the age group between 30 to 35 is better aware of this HIV/AIDS than the other age groups. Now we can infer that middle aged people have a better awareness than the other age groups and the urban population is more aware of this disease than the rural population.

II. Education

It is a common belief that if the individual is educated his/her awareness is greater and deeper on various fields of life. Obviously their awareness and knowledge about HIV/AIDS through media becomes easier for them. Education helps one to know how to protect himself/herself from the virus. The general hypothetical assumption is higher the education of the respondents, greater the level of awareness of the sickness through media. Having this at the backdrop the researcher analyses the area of awareness among the Self Help Groups.

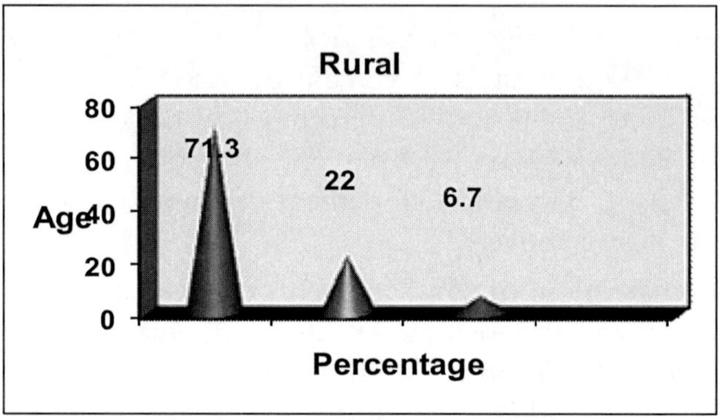

Description	Respondent	Percentage
Below 10th std	107	71.3
+2	33	22.0
UG	10	6.7
Total	**150**	**100.0**

It is amazing to note that 71.3 per cent of the respondents did have done their schooling below 10th Standard. 22 per cent of them have completed their higher secondary. This is followed by 6.7 per cent who have done their UG level.

It is to be noted that majority that is 71.3 per cent of the respondents had a low educational background. This adds to the analysis why most of them are under the below poverty line category.

Description	Respondent	Percentage
Below 1oth	114	76.0
Higher secondary	14	9.3
Undergraduate	11	7.3
Post graduate	6	4.0
others	5	3.3
Total	**150**	**100**

Describe that76% people are below the category of 10th std. 9.3%have done their higher secondary level education 7.3 %have done their undergraduate. 4% of people have done their post graduate and 3.3% have done some other studies.

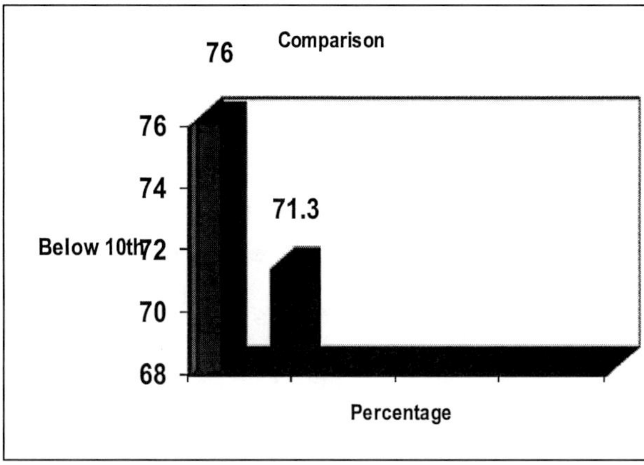

When studied about the educational background it is noticed that in rural areas people who have studied up to std 10 is 71.3 and in the urban areas it is 76%. It looks contradictory that in urban areas the percentage of people with 10th std qualification is more than the rural areas. But the general educational standards are higher in urban areas.

III. Occupation

The researcher feels that a sound income helps family to meet its basic needs thereby creating a feeling of important about family and its values. Media plays a significant role among those who earn more. They have easy access to the media and thus the level of awareness is higher.

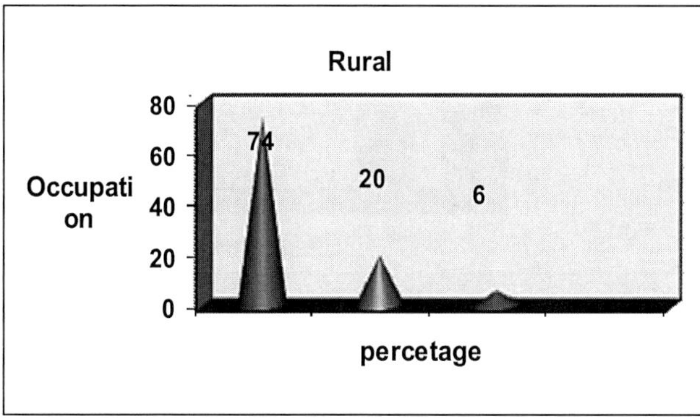

Description	Respondent	Percentage
Coolie	111	74.0
PVT	30	20.0
GOVT	9	6.0
Total	**150**	**100.0**

It can be seen from the table 74 per cent of the respondents are from the daily wage category (coolie). Only 6 per cent fall under the Government employment. While 20 per cent of them are busy with their private work.

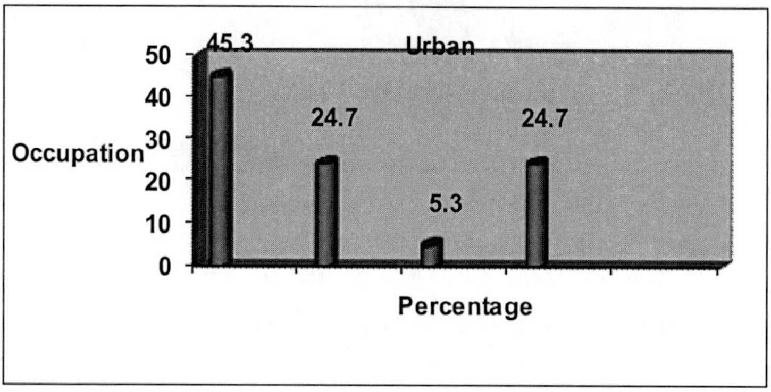

Description	Respondent	Percentage
Coolie	68	45.3
Private	37	24.7
Government	8	5.3
Own	37	24.7
Total	**150**	**100**

Explains that 45.3% people are still going for coolie work. 24.7 people are doing private jobs. 24.7% people have their own work and 5.3% people are doing government job.

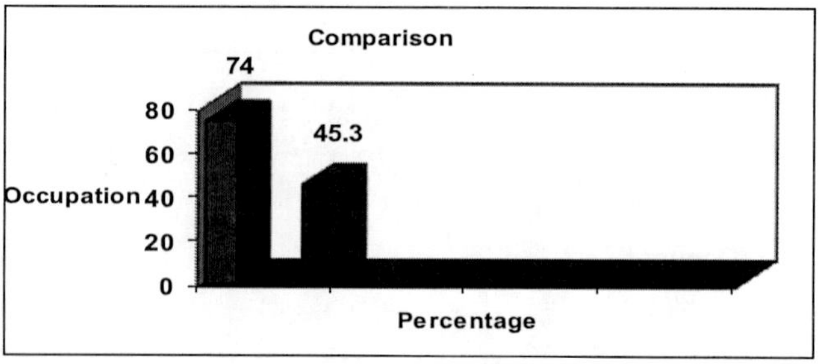

It is quite obvious to notice that nearly 74% of the people are daily wage earners in rural areas and 45.3% are there in the urban areas. It is only natural that the rural areas have not that much industry to attract more workers in the organized sector.

IV. Income

Families that are not able to meet their end become dysfunctional families. The risk of getting into any sickness is higher among the lower income groups. Normally it is the income that divides the families according to their earning capacity. In many of the corporate firms, even the employees are given quarters according to the earning capacity such as Lower Income Group, Middle Income Group and Higher Income Group. It measures the standard of living in most of the societies. Accordingly the level of awareness differs.

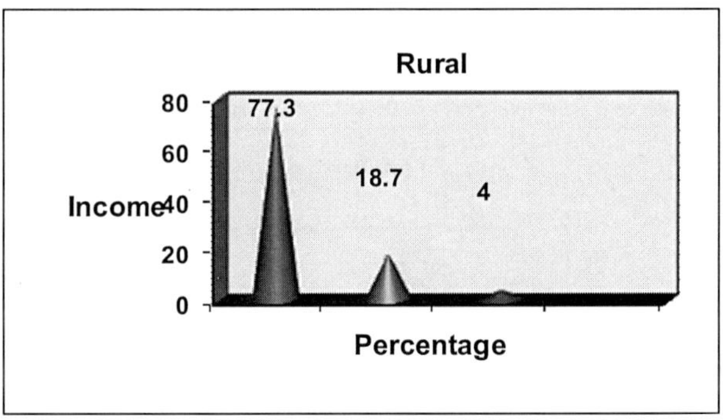

Description	Respondent	Percentage
below 1000	116	77.3
1000-2000	28	18.7
2000-3000	6	4.0
Total	**150**	**100.0**

The above table shows the earnings of the respondents. It is seen that 77 percent of respondents are below Rs. 1000 category and 18.7 percent of them have family income from Rs. 1000 to 2000. Interestingly only mere 4 percent are earning between 2000 to 3000.

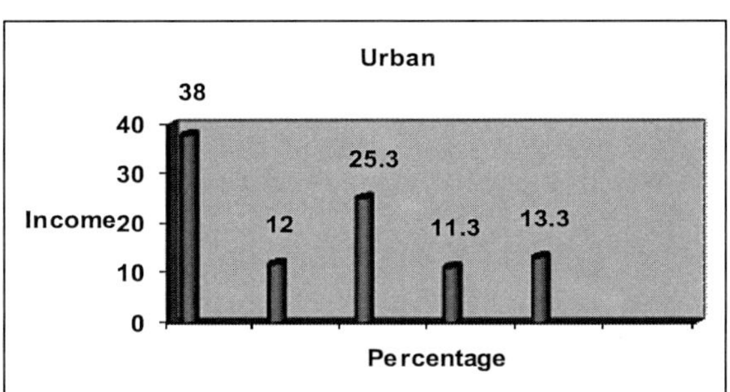

DESCRIPTION	RESPONDENT	PERCENTAGE
Below 1000	57	38.0
1000-2000	18	12.0
2000-3000	38	25.3
3000-4000	17	11.3
4000-5000	20	13.3
Total	**150**	**100**

illustrates that even in city 23% of people are living under poverty line. 25.3% people earn Rs 2000 – 3000 per month. 13.3% people earn Rs 4000-5000 per month; 12% of people earn Rs 1000-2000 and 11.3% people earn 3000-4000 per month.

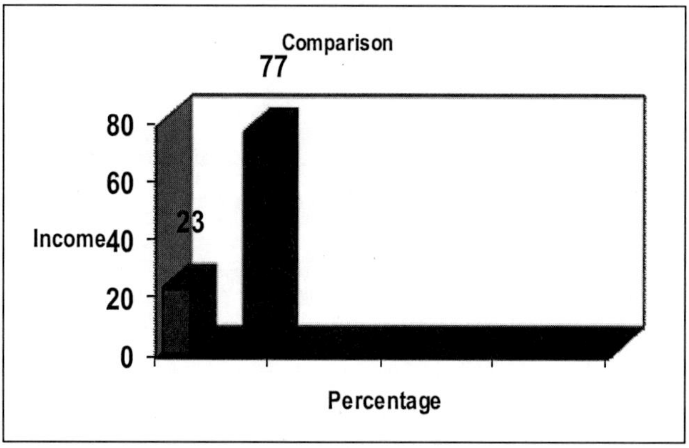

Based on occupational pattern we learn that 23% of the urban people live below poverty line where as in rural areas more than double the percentage i.e. 77% live below poverty line. They earn less than 1000 rupees per month. In the all India level only 22% of people live below poverty line but it differs from region to region.

V. Family Members

Family plays a significant role in the social set up of our country. Family can bring all the values together and live it. Disintegrated families also can play havoc in the social value system. Family is the first basic unit in an individual's life. Traditionally the needs of the family members were met by the institution of family the one where the basic needs were provided for.

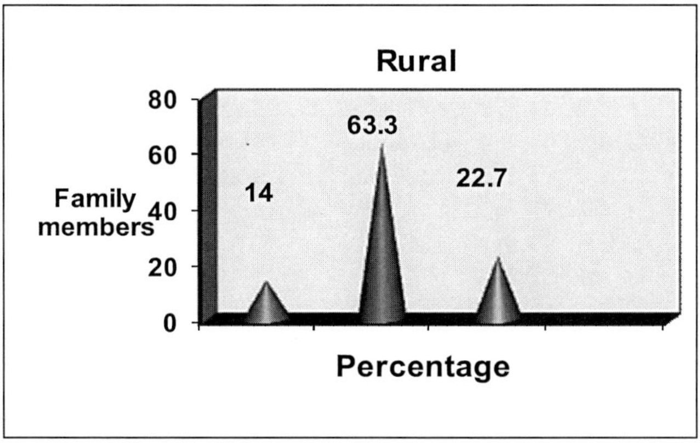

Description	Respondent	Percentage
Below 3	21	14.0
3-5	95	63.3
5 and above	34	22.7
Total	**150**	**100.0**

According to Table – 5 we see that 14 percent come under below 3 marking. 63. 3 percent fall under 3 to 5 marking. Only 22. 7 come under 5 and above marking level.

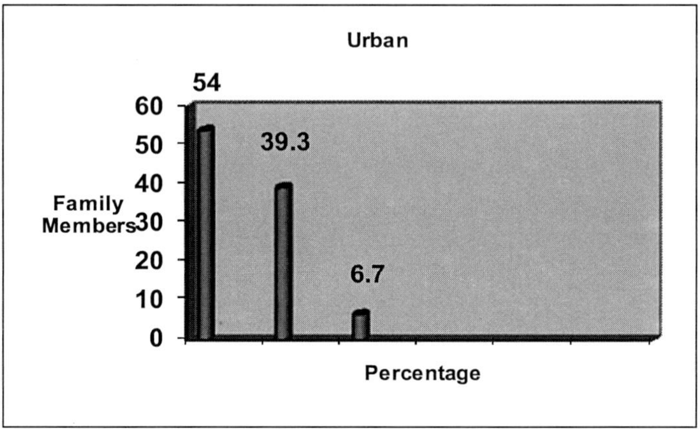

Description	Respondent	Percentage
Below3	81	54.0
3-5	59	39.3
Above5	10	6.7
Total	**150**	**100**

Shows that 54% have less than 3 members in a family.39.3% family have three to five members in a family. Only 6.7% people have more than five members in a family.

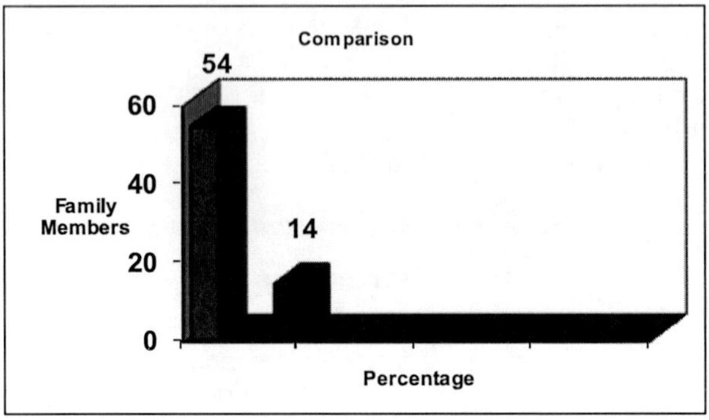

Coming to the point of family members it is noticed that the number of members in family with three or less is 54% of the families in urban areas, and in rural areas it is only 14%. This may be due to lack of education and other factors like income

Awareness on Hiv/Aids

Awareness occurs within the society and built upon existing processes at all levels. All the Government and Non-Government agencies are involved mostly in awareness programme. Every awareness gets into the root cause of the issue and eventually becomes an educative channel.

Hence, the researcher has analyzed the seriousness of the disease – HIV through Awareness concept in his design of the thesis. Keeping awareness as its first step the researcher has dealt deeply into various aspects of HIV/AIDS.

1. What do you understand by HIV or AIDS?

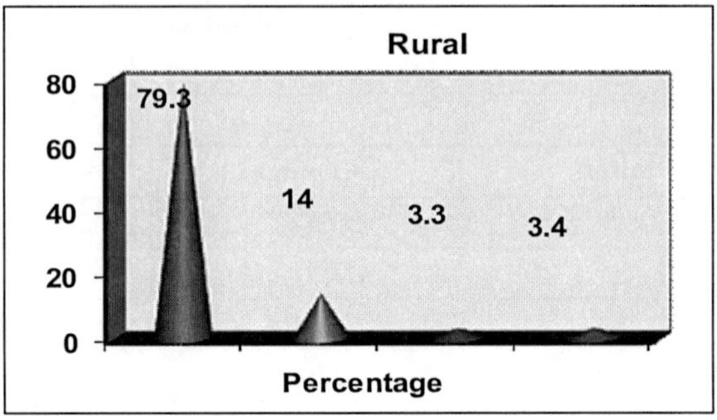

Table No: 1

Description	Respondent	Percentage
It is a very serious sickness	119	79.3
It kills many people	21	14.0
I do not know the seriousness	5	3.3
I know nothing about it	5	3.4
Total	**150**	**100.0**

The above mentioned table shows that 79.3% of respondents knew that HIV/AIDS is a very serious disease. 14% of respondents say that HIV/AIDS kills many people and 3.3% respondents answer that they do not know the seriousness of the disease and only 3.4% have not heard anything about HIV/AIDS.

The large number of respondents does know that HIV/AIDS is a very serious disease.

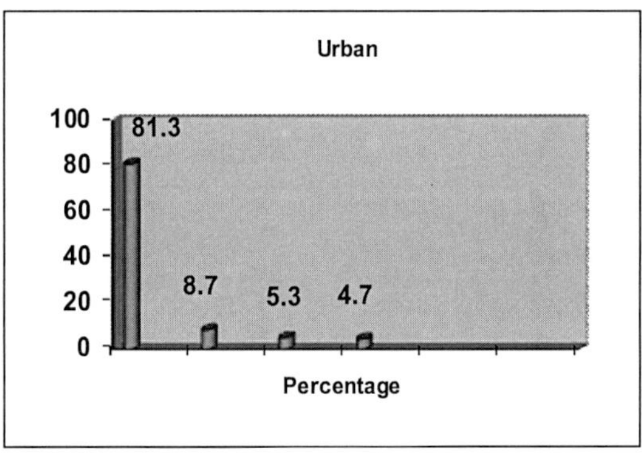

Description	Respondent	Percentage
It is a very serious sickness.	122	81.3
It kills many people.	13	8.7
I do not know the seriousness.	8	5.3
I know nothing.	7	4.7
Total	**150**	**100**

Points out that 81.3% people are aware that HIV/AIDS is a serious disease. 8.7% people know that it kills many people. 5.3% feel that they do not know the seriousness of the disease. Only 4.7% people do not know anything about the seriousness of the disease.

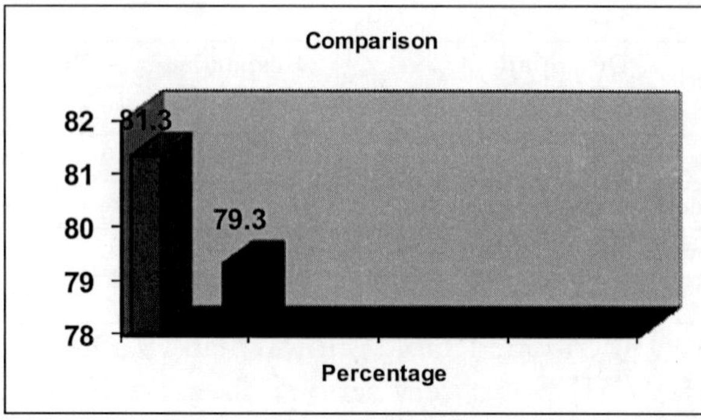

It is heartening to note that nearly 81.3% in urban area and 79.3% in rural areas know that HIV/AIDS is a very serious disease and it is an important factor that may prevent the diseases from spreading one person to the other. This makes the people conscious of the risks of this disease.

2. HIV/AIDS is caused by

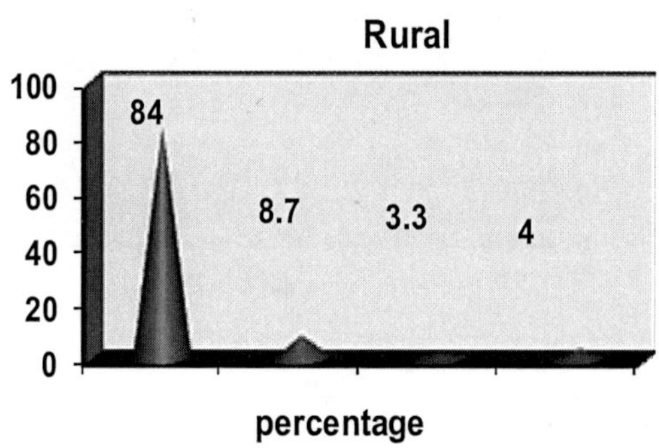

Table No: 2

Description	Respondent	percentage
Virus	126	84.0
Bacteria	13	8.7
Fungus	5	3.3
Don't know	6	4.0
Total	**150**	**100**

This table explains that 84% of respondent said that the HIV/AIDS spreads through virus. 8.7% of respondent said that the HIV/AIDS spreads through bacteria. 3.3% of people said it spreads through fungus, and 4% people do not have any idea about what causes HIV/AIDS.

From the above table I understand that the majority of respondent knew that HIV/AIDS spreads through virus.

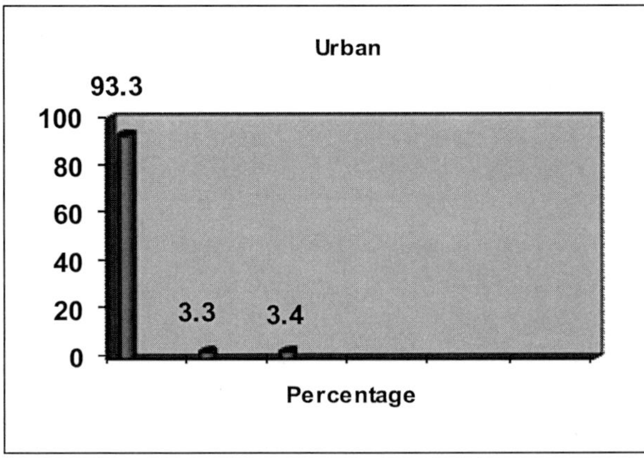

Description	Respondent	Percentage
Virus	140	93.3
Bacteria	5	3.3
Don't know	5	3.4
Total	**150**	**100**

From the above table 93.3% of people answered that virus is the cause for the HIV/AIDS, and 3.4% of people responded Bacteria and 3.4% people answered that they do not know the cause for HIV/AIDS.

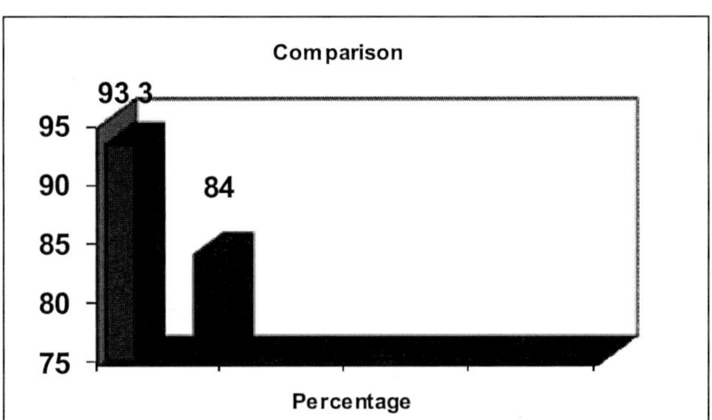

Nearly 93.3% of the urban people and 84% of the rural people have understood that it is caused by virus. It is a welcome symptom. This may be a scientific thing but it is a vital point regarding this disease.

3. HIV/AIDS is a problem of homosexual

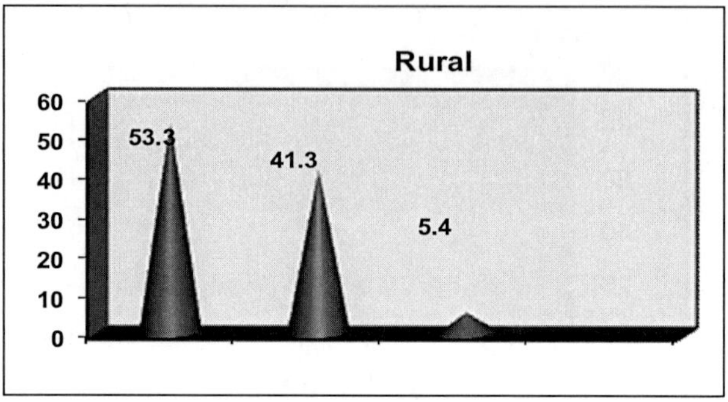

Table No: 3

Description	Respondent	Percentage
yes	80	53.3
No	62	41.3
Don't know	8	5.3
Total	**150**	**100**

53.3% of respondents says that HIV/AIDS is a homosexual, 41.35 of respondent say 41.3% people say that it is not a problem of homosexual and 5.4% respondent say that they do not know anything about this sickness.

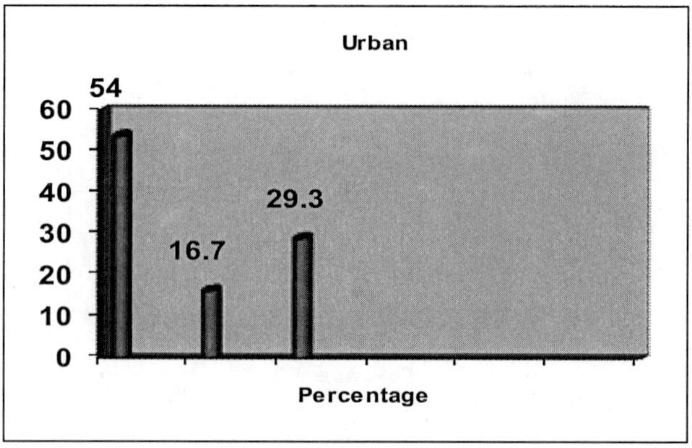

Description	Respondent	Percentage
Yes	81	54.0
No	25	16.7
Don't know	44	29.3
Total	**150**	**100**

When the question was asked whether HIV/AIDS is a problem of homosexuals 54% of the people responded yes; 16.7% of people responded no and 29.3% of people had no idea.

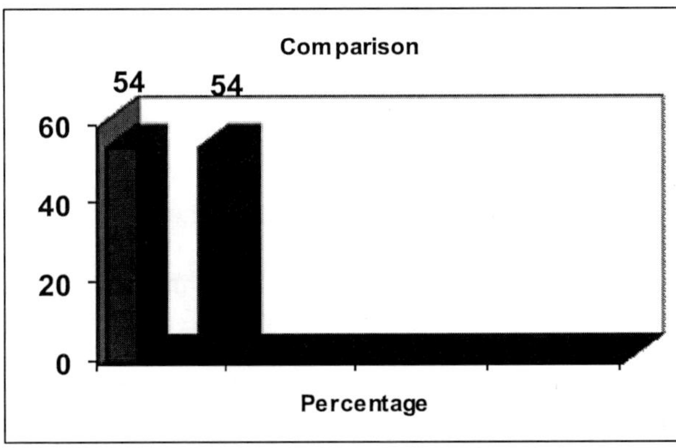

It is surprising to note that nearly 54% of the rural and urban populations consider it as a problem of homosexuals. This is a very peculiar thing strange to our country but it is quite encouraging that many people know about it.

4. In your opinion what is the worst killer disease in our country?

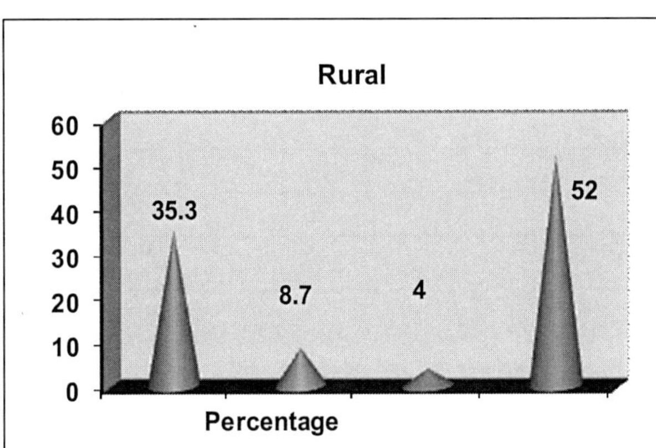

Table No: 4

Description	Respondent	Percentage
Cancer	53	35.3
TB	13	8.7
Heart disease	6	4.0
HIV/AIDS	78	52.0
Total	**150**	**100**

The answers for the above questions, 52% of the people feel that the worst killer in our country is HIV/AIDS; 35.3%people sense the worse killer in our country is cancer; 8.7% people feel that TB is the worst killer in our country, and 4% people feel that the worst killer is none other than the heart disease.

The majority of people feel that the worst killer is the HIV/AIDS.

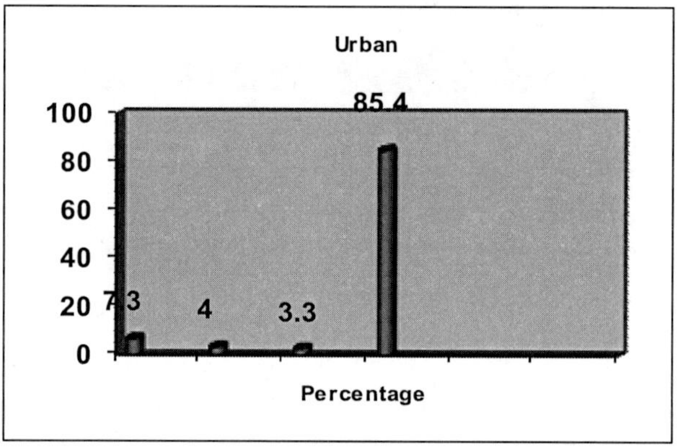

Description	Respondent	Percentage
Cancer	11	7.3
TB	6	4.0
Heart disease	5	3.3
HIV/AIDS	128	85.4
Total	**150**	**100**

The worst killer disease in our country for 7.3% of the people said that it is none other than cancer, 4% of the people suggested that it is TB, 3.3% of the people said that it is heart diseases and the majority i.e. 85.4% of the people responded that it is HIV/AIDS.

It is remarkable to note that the majority i.e. 85.3% of people have the right knowledge of the terrific disease HIV/AIDS and opted for it as the worst killer disease in our country.

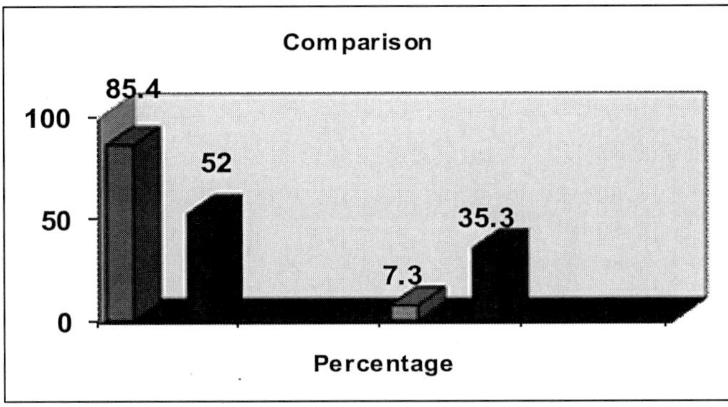

There is a vast difference of opinion between the rich and the poor in identifying the worst killer disease in our country. While 85.4 of the urban people opine that HIV/AIDS is the worst killer, only 52% of rural folk consider it as the same. Another interesting thing is nearly 35.3% of the rural folk consider cancer as the worst killing disease whereas only 7.3 % of the urban people consider it as the same.

5. As for as HIV/ AIDS is concerned, what is its status in India?

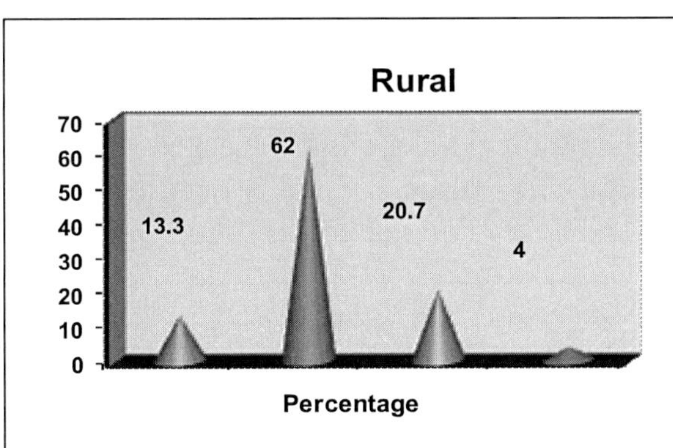

Table No: 5

Description	Respondent	Percentage
First	20	13.3
Second	93	62.0
Third	31	20.7
Any other	6	4.0
Total	**150**	**100**

As for as HIV/AIDS is concerned 62% respondents said that India ranks second place in the world, 20.7% respondents said that India is in third place, 13.3% respondents said that India is in first place, and 4% said they do not know in which place India stands.

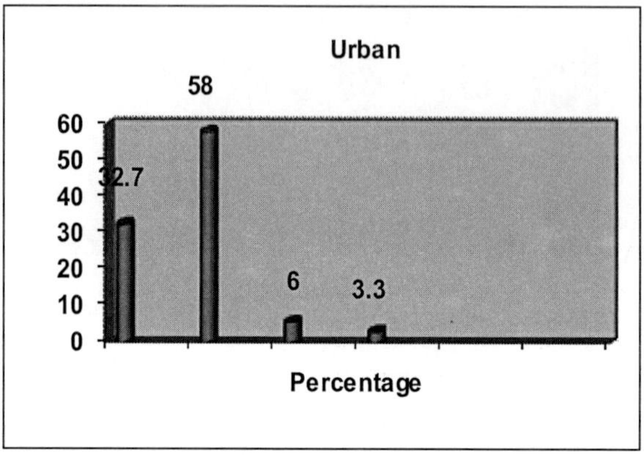

Description	Respondent	Percentage
First	49	32.7
Second	87	58.0
Third	9	6.0
Any other	5	3.3
Total	**150**	**100**

The status of India regarding to the concept of HIV 58% of people answered that India possess the second place, 32.7% of the people opined that India is in the first place, 6% of people answered that India is in the third place and 3.3% of the people had no idea about the place India possesses as for as the HIV is concerned.

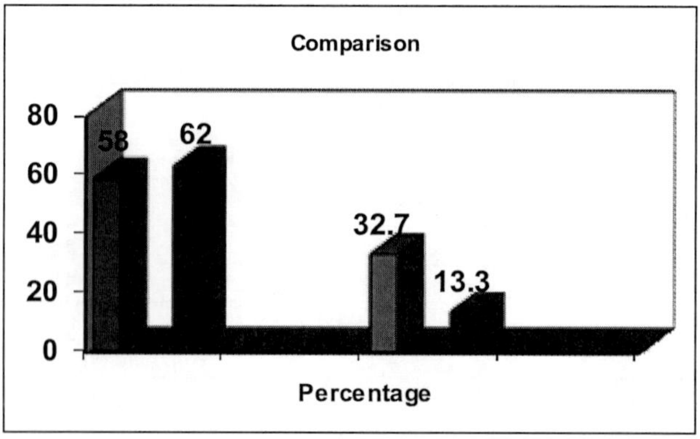

Nearly 58% of the urban population and 62% of the rural population think that India stands second in the HIV/AIDS disease position. 32.7% of the urban and 13.3 % of rural that India ranks first in this killer disease. Really though India ranks second in the world population wise most number of HIV/AIDS affected people are in India.

6. What are the symptoms?

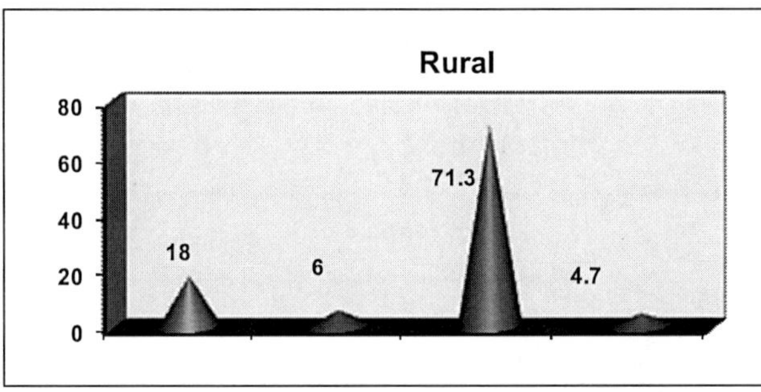

Table No: 6

Description	Respondent	Percentage
Fever	27	18.0
Tiredness	9	6.0
Loss of weight	107	71.3
Not feeling hungry	7	4.7
Total	**150**	**100**

The symptoms for HIV/AIDS for 71.3% is loss of weight, for 18% of respondents it is fever, 6% say that tiredness is the, and 4.7% of the people say that the symptom is not feeling hungry. The majority of the people feel that loss of weight is the main symptom.

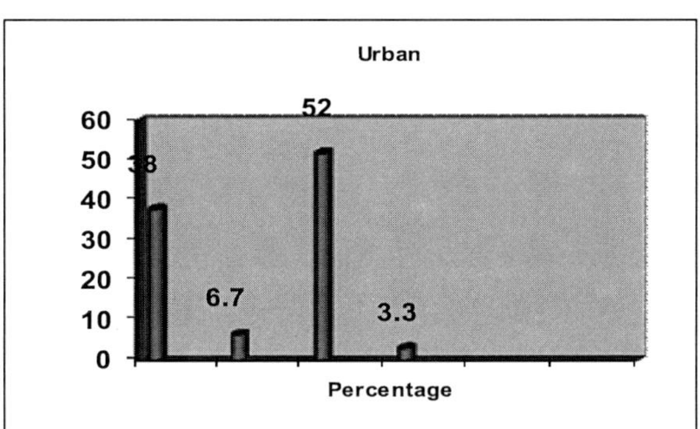

Description	Respondent	Percentage
Fever	57	38.0
Tiredness	10	6.7
Loss of weight	78	52.0
Not feeling hungry	5	3.3
Total	**150**	**100**

The symptoms for HIV/AIDS for 52% of people is none other than loss of weight, for 38% of people it is fever, 6.7% of people it is tiredness and 3.3% of people responded the symptoms for HIV/AIDS is not feeling hungry.

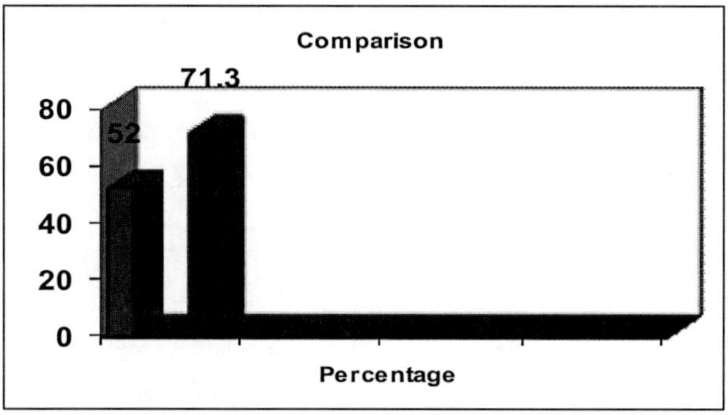

It is surprising to note that 52% of the urban population and 71.3% of the rural population have understood that loss of weight is the main symptoms of HIV/AIDS. Though this is a medical perception, even ordinary people have known this aspect.

7. I became deeply aware of the Problems of HIV/Aids through

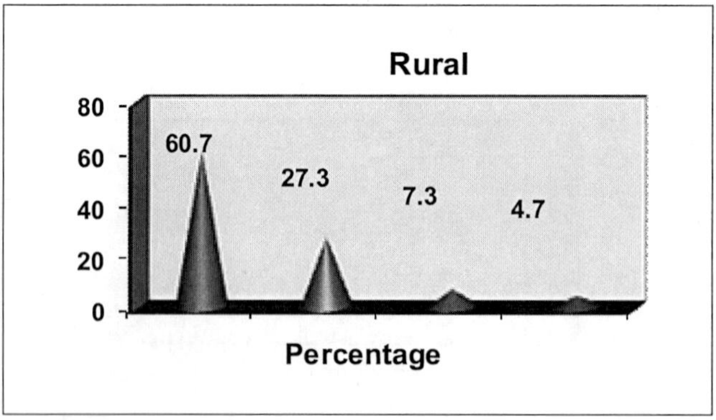

Table No: 7

Description	Respondent	Percentage
TV programmes	91	60.7
Radio	41	27.3
Movies	11	7.3
Any other	7	4.7
Total	**150**	**100**

60.7% respondent said that they received HIV/AIDS information from TV, 27.3% said they received information from radio, 7.3% respondent said that they came to know about HIV/AIDS movies, and 4.7%respondent came to know about through HIV/AIDS through other means.

Among the media TV the audio video medium has more influence among people. From the above table it is clear that 60.7% people came to know about HIV/AIDS through this powerful medium.

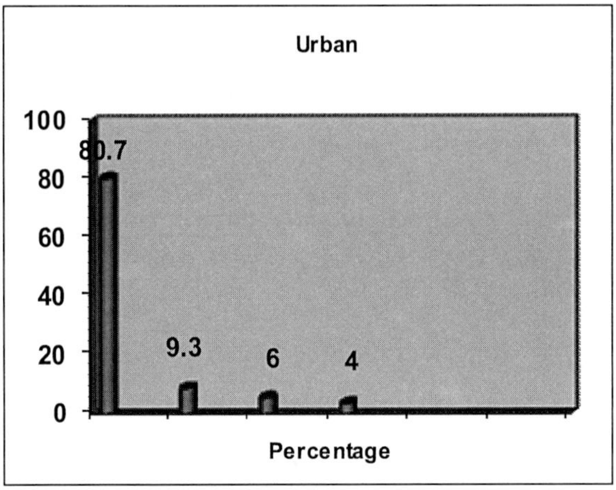

Description	Respondent	Percentage
TV programme	121	80.7
Radio	14	9.3
Movies	9	6.0
Any other	6	4.0
Total	150	100

A large number of 80.7% of people are deeply aware of the problems of HIV/AIDS through the TV programmes, 9.3% of people came to know through the means of radio, 6% of people responded with the medium of movies, and 4% of people had the idea of other than the above three options.

Notably to say that 80.7% of people became deeply aware of the problems of HIV/AIDS through TV programmes.

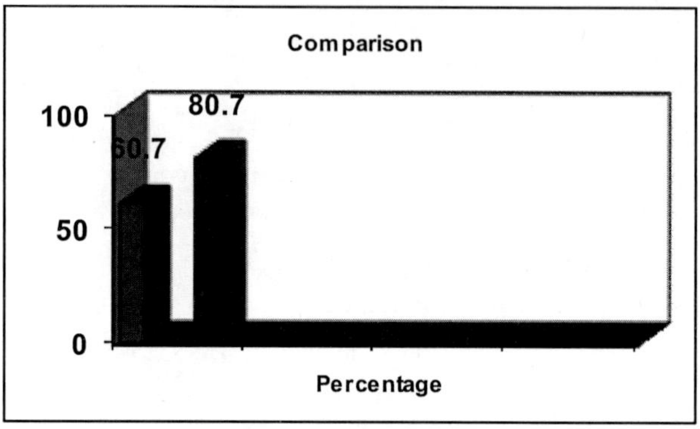

The highest percentage of population (both rural 60.7% and urban 80.7%) agree that they came to know about HIV/AIDS through Television. This shows the importance of TV in creating awareness. In fact among the means of media television ranks first in India why even in the world.

8. Do you know how long a person will live with AIDS?

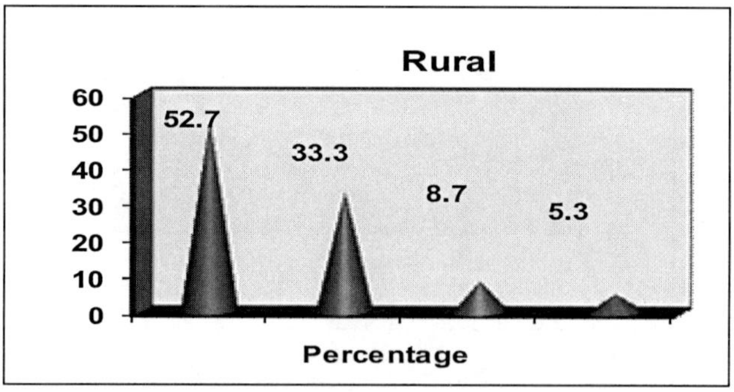

Table No: 8

Description	Respondent	Percentage
Approximately 5 years	79	52.7
Approximately 10 years	50	33.3
Approximately 15 years	13	8.7
Do not know	8	5.3
Total	**150**	**100**

From this mentioned table the concept of people on how long a person will live with AIDS is said as for 52.7% HIV/AIDS patient will live for five years, 33.3% will live for ten years, 8.7% will live for fifteen years, and 5.3% people have no idea for how long these patients will live.

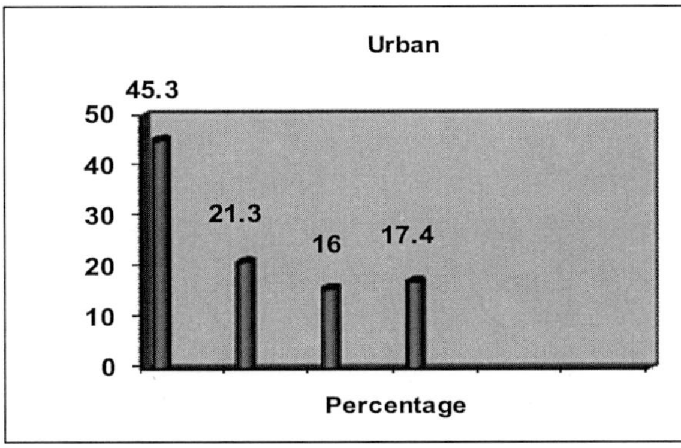

Description	Respondent	Percentage
Approximately 5 years	68	45.3
Approximately 10 years	32	21.3
Approximately 15 years	24	16.0
Don't know	26	17.4
Total	**150**	**100**

The response for the above question 45.3% of people said that approximately 5 years a person will live with AIDS, 21.3% of people answered that approximately 10 years, 16% of people said that approximately 15 years, and 17.4 % were not aware of the time a person will live with AIDS.

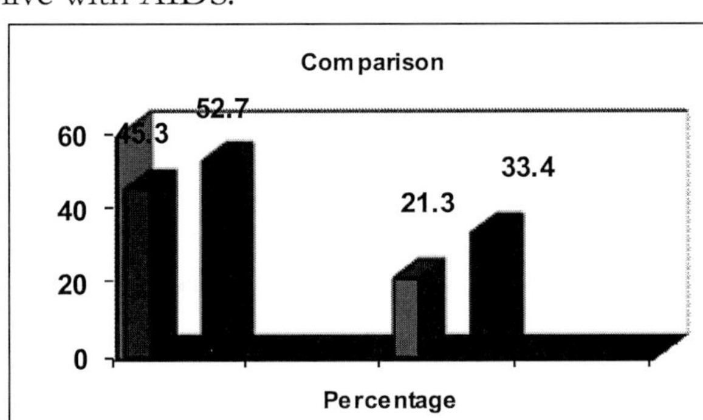

When we posed the question of longevity of the HIV/AIDS infected patients 52.7% the rural people say that they may approximately live for 5 years where as only 45.3% urban people accept this theory. 21.3% of urban people say that patients can live for 10 years but 33.3% of the rural people say that the patients can live for 10 years. These statements may be elusive as we have no concrete proofs to prove this longevity.

9. In what Way could we use the Media in a Better way to bring about more awareness?

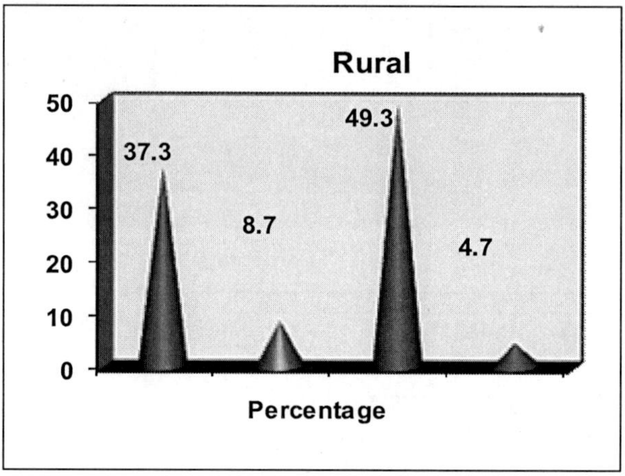

Table No: 9

Description	Respondent	Percentage
Discussion	56	37.3
Open sharing	13	8.7
Preventive care and counseling centre	74	49.3
Do not know	7	4.7
Total	**150**	**100**

49.3% respondent feel that media could bring better awareness through counseling centers. 37.3% respondents feel that through discussion media could bring more awareness. 8.7% respondents feel that through open sharing it would be better informed. And 4.7% people do not know about media awareness.

More of 40.3% people feel through preventive care and counseling centre better information could be given.

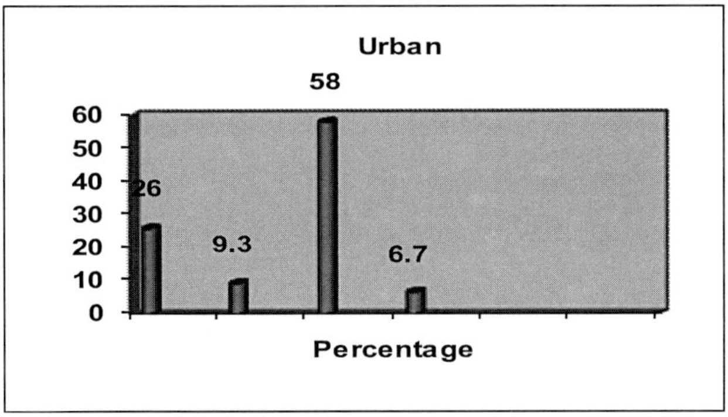

Description	Respondent	Percentage
Discussion	39	26.0
Open sharing	14	9.3
Preventive care &counseling	87	58.0
Don't know	10	6.7
Total	**150**	**100**

58% of people responded that best way we can use the media in a better way to bring about more awareness is preventive care counseling centre, 26% of people felt that the apt way for the awareness for the AIDS is through discussion, 9.3% of the people were on the side of open sharing and 6.7% of people were unaware of any way to bring about more awareness.

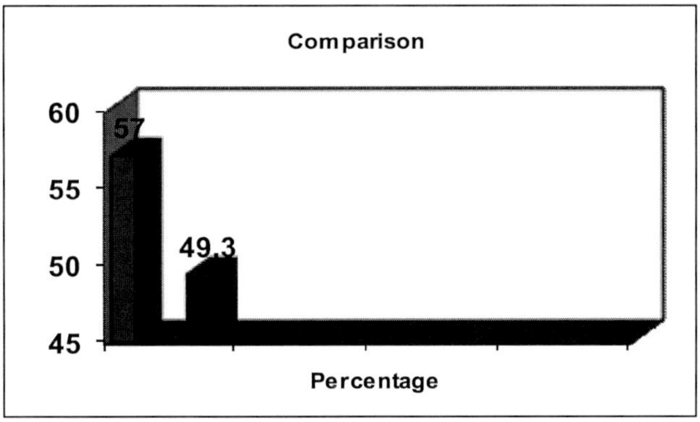

Many are of the opinion that more awareness should be created about the preventive care and counseling aspects of the disease. The difference between the rural (49.3%) and the urban (57%) is not much. Hence it is understood that the preventive aspect of the disease should be stressed more by the media. Now all the schemes focus their attention more on the preventive side than on the curative side.

10. In your knowledge, how does Media project the Spread of Virus?

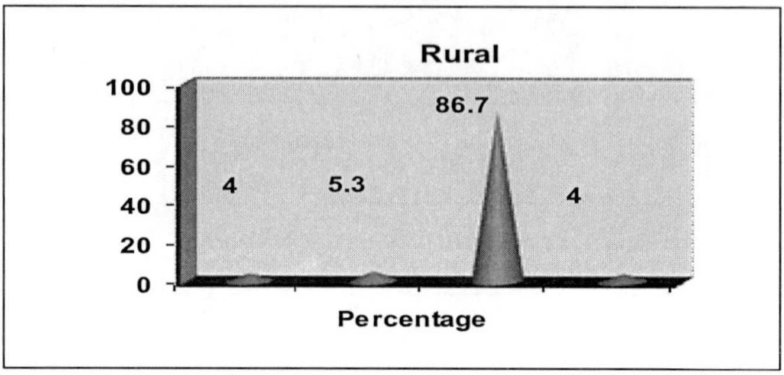

Table No: 10

Description	Respondent	Percentage
Sharing of clothes	6	4.0
Pregnant mother to child	8	5.3
Unsafe sex	130	86.7
Infected blood	6	4.0
Total	**150**	**100**

From the above table 86.7% say that media project the spread of virus through unsafe sex, 5.3% say that media project the spread of virus through pregnant mother to child. 4% say that media project the spread of virus through sharing of clothes and 4% through infected blood.

The majority of people say that the projection of spread of virus through unsafe sex.

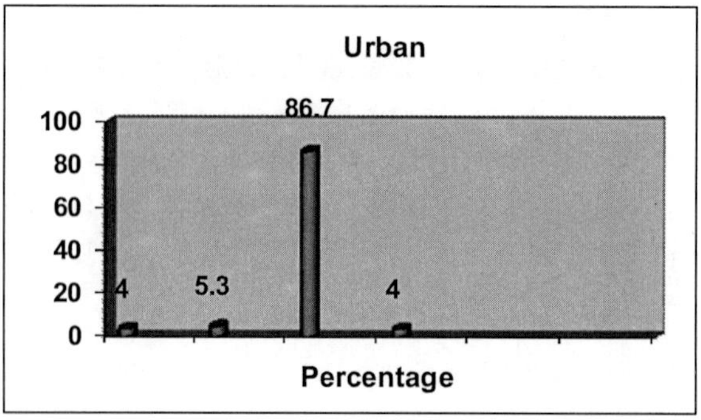

Description	Respondent	Percentage
Sharing of clothes	6	4.0
Pregnant mother to child	8	5.3
Unsafe sex	130	86.7
Infected blood	6	4.0
Total	**150**	**100**

From the above table it is said that 86.7% of respondent say that they received knowledge from the media through unsafe sex the virus is spreading, whereas 5.3% of respondent say through pregnant mother to the child. Only 4% of respondent say that the virus spread through infected blood and sharing of clothes.

It is important to note that majority of 86.7% people know the cause is through unsafe sex.

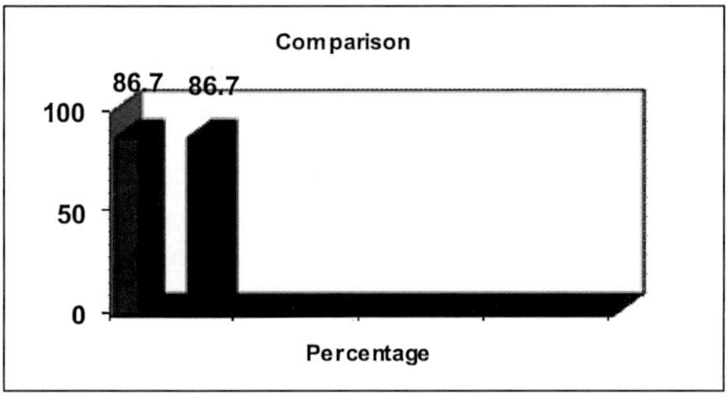

From the media people became aware that unsafe sex is the main cause for the spreading of HIV/AIDS. It is really surprising to note that both rural (86.7%) and urban (86.7%) percentages are the same and the media has done a good job in creating awareness among the people. This aspect should be stressed further by the media. So that many people are saved from this dreadful disease.

11. Have you Learnt form Media that HIV Spreads from Mother to Child?

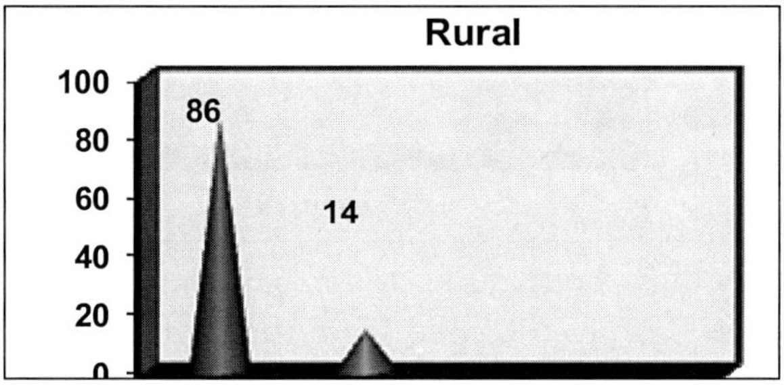

Table No: 11

Description	Respondent	Percentage
Yes	129	86.0
No	21	14.0
Total	**150**	**100**

86% of respondent say that they learnt from media that HIV/AIDS spreads from mother to child, and 14% of respondent learnt from media that HIV/AIDS does not spread from mother to child.

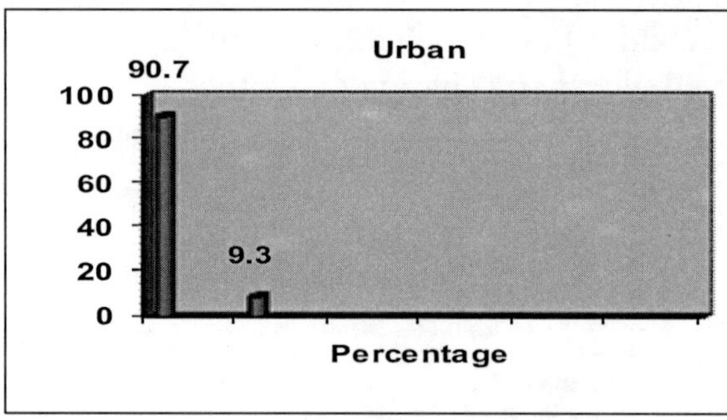

Description	Respondent	Percentage
Yes	136	90.7
no	14	9.3
Total	**150**	**100**

90.7% of people learnt form media that HIV spreads from mother to child, and only 9.3% of people deny the above affirmation that they learnt from media that HIV spreads from mother to child.

It is admiring fact that 90.7% of the people learnt form media that HIV spreads from mother to child.

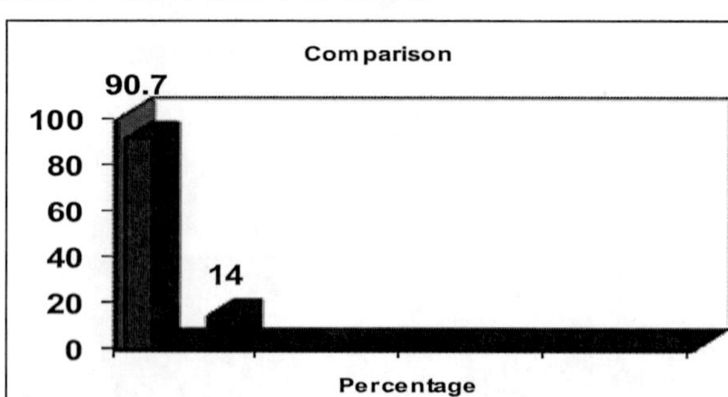

The media has been able to make the people aware that HIV/AIDS passes on to the child from the mother. Nearly 90.7% of urban people and 86% of rural people believe this. But in rural areas nearly 14% of the people do not believe this as a possibility. This concept may be stressed by the social workers who are working with the HIV/AIDS affected mothers.

12. Media educate that if you take the drug Navarapin, the child will not be affected by HIV/AIDS.

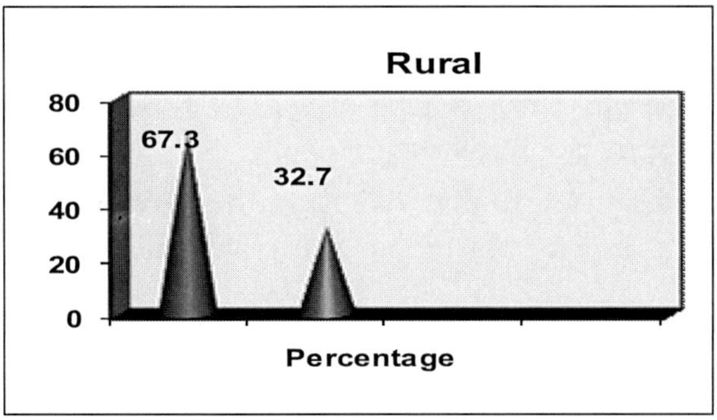

Table No: 12

Description	Respondent	Percentage
Yes	101	67.3
No	49	32.7
Total	**150**	**100**

67.3% respondent say that media educates that if they take the drug Navarapin the child may not be affected by HIV/AIDS, while 32.7% respondents say that if they take Navarapin also the child may get HIV/AIDS.

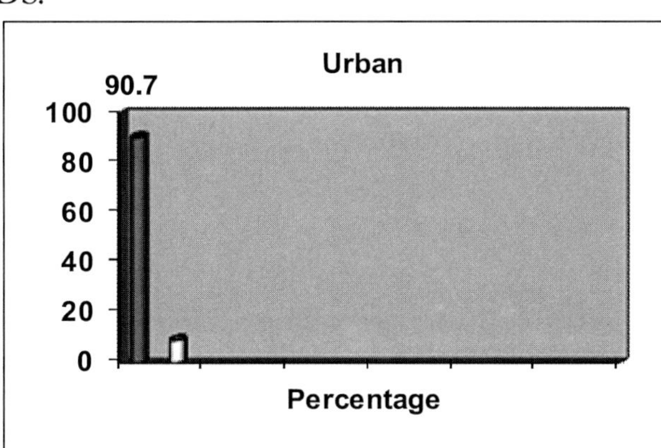

Description	Respondent	Percentage
Yes	136	90.7
No	14	9.3
Total	**150**	**100**

90.7% of the people strongly affirm to the view points of the media that it educates, taking the drug Navarapin the child will not be affected by HIV/AIDS, while on the other hand 9.3% of the people disagree that the child will not be affected by HIV/AIDS by taking the drug Navarapin taught by the media.

It is interesting to note that 90.7% of the people agree that media educate taking the drug Navarapin the child will not be affected by HIV/AIDS.

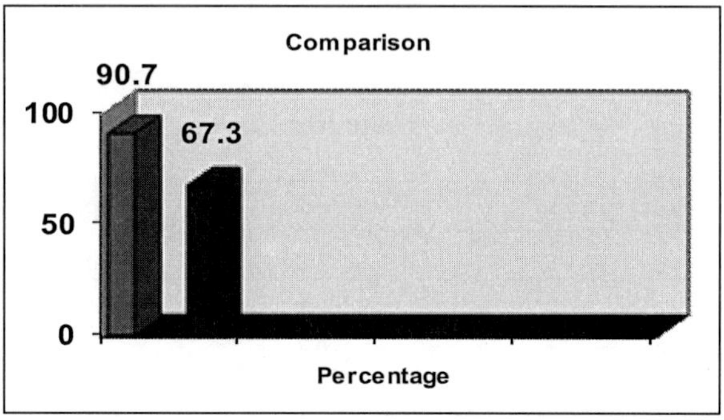

The introduction of Navarapin can prevent HIV/AIDS spreading to the child from the mother is known to many people both rural and urban. Since in urban areas the media facilities are more nearly 90.7% know about this, where as in rural areas only 67.3% know about it. The use of this medicine should be widely propagated to make pregnant mothers to use this medicine.

Media Information Source

Sharing knowledge, experiences and good practice is a key way to improve the effectiveness of all organizations involved in the response to the HIV/AIDS. Today the media plays a significant role and provides a lot of material to educate people and thus reduce the calamity of HIV/AIDS. The media has a pivotal role to play in the AIDS response. Now 25 years into the epidemic, public understanding of how HIV is prevented and treated is mixed, and basic awareness about AIDS and its impact is sorely lacking in many parts of the world, particularly among women and children. With its wide-reaching, global infrastructure and communications expertise, the media's ability to change the course of the AIDS crisis is virtually unparalleled. We know a lot more about this sickness now than we did then. It is mainly by media influence and its sources. Media brings forward appropriate message that the important thing is to ensure that people in the affected groups know that it is important to act in ways that are likely to keep them safe. Today people have got into a sense of the serious killer now than 20 years ago. Hence, this study brings forward the role of media in bringing out awareness among the target groups of Keechalam and Saidapet.

13. What are the Different Forms of Media you have in your House?

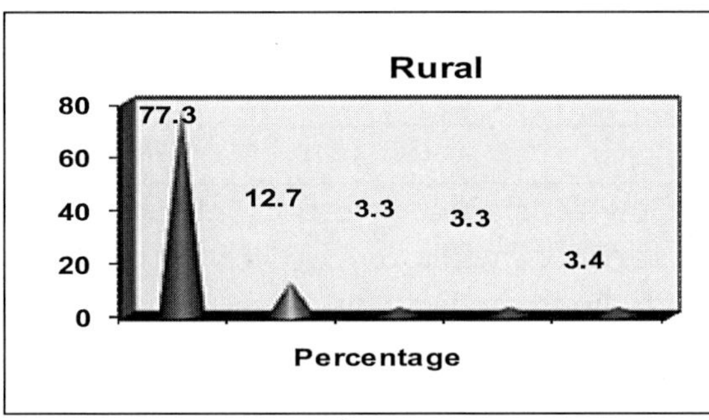

Table No: 13

Description	Respondent	Percentage
TV	116	77.3
Radio	19	12.7
News paper	5	3.3
Magazine	5	3.4
Any other	5	3.4
Total	**150**	**100**

According to the above table, 77.3% of people have TV in their house, 12.7% of people have radio in their house, 3.3% of people have magazine, newspaper and 3.4 % other medium in their house.

The majority of the people own TV in their house.

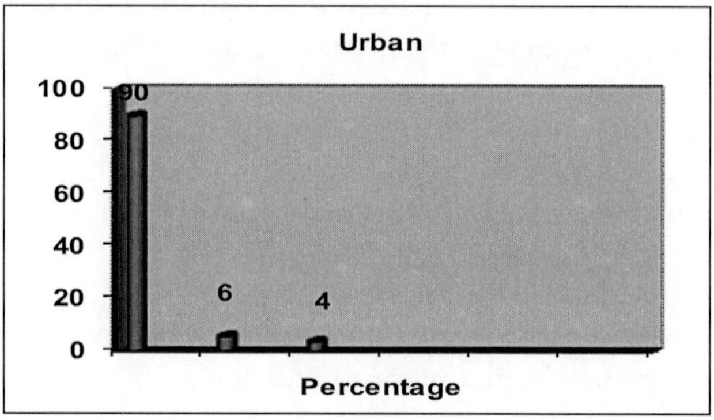

Description	Respondent	Percentage
TV	135	90.0
Radio	9	6.0
News paper	6	4.0
Total	**150**	**100**

The answer for the mentioned question 90% of the people felt that TV is the best form of media they found in their house, 6% of the people said that radio is the best for of media they found in their house and 4% of the people felt that newspaper is the best medium they found in their house.

The majority of 90% of people opt for TV as the best form of media they have in their house.

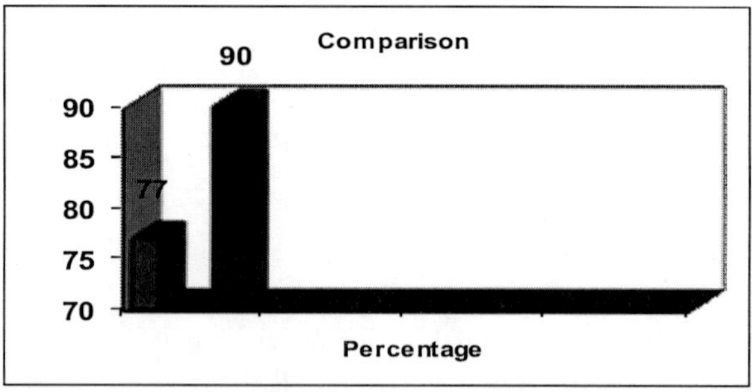

The importance of television in providing information about HIV/AIDS should be taken note of by all. In the urban areas nearly 90% and in the rural areas nearly 77.3% possess television sets. This is really a notable feature in a poor country like India. The number of television sets should be increased in the rural areas.

14. I came to know the Most about HIV/AIDS through

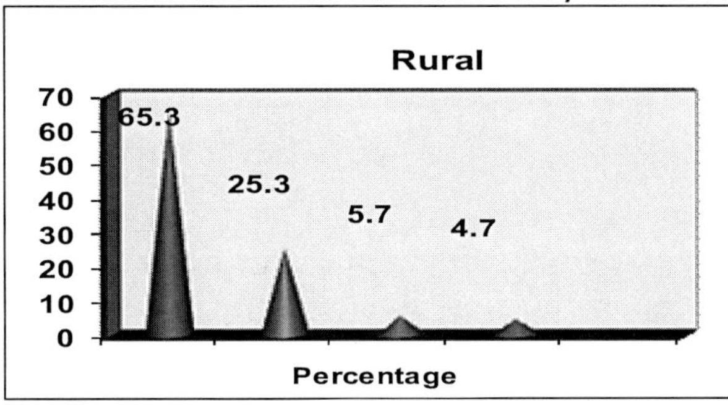

Table No: 14

Description	Respondent	Percentage
TV	98	65.3
Radio	38	25.3
Newspaper	8	5.1
Magazine	6	4.3
Total	**150**	**100**

The answer for the above question 65.3% of people responded TV is the medium through which they came to know the most about HIV/AIDS, 25.3% of people came to know the most about HIV/AIDS through radio, 5.1% of people responded newspaper as their means, 4.3% of people came to know through magazine.

TV is the main medium through which the people came to know the most about HIV/AIDS.

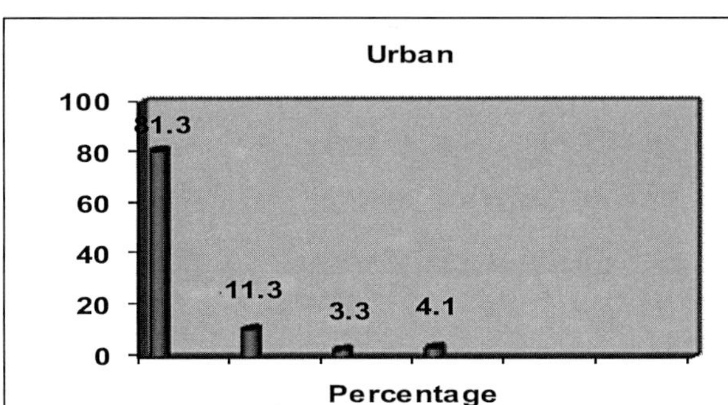

Description	Respondent	Percentage
TV	122	81.3
Radio	17	11.3
Newspaper	5	3.3
Magazine	6	4.1
Total	**150**	**100**

A very good number of 81.3% of people came to know the most about HIV/AIDS through TV, 11.3% of the people got the awareness about HIV/AIDS through the means of radio, 4.1% of the people got to know through magazine, and only 3.3% of the people came to know the most about HIV/AIDS through newspaper.

It is necessary to point out that the large number of 81.3% of the people came to know the most about HIV/AIDS through the means of TV.

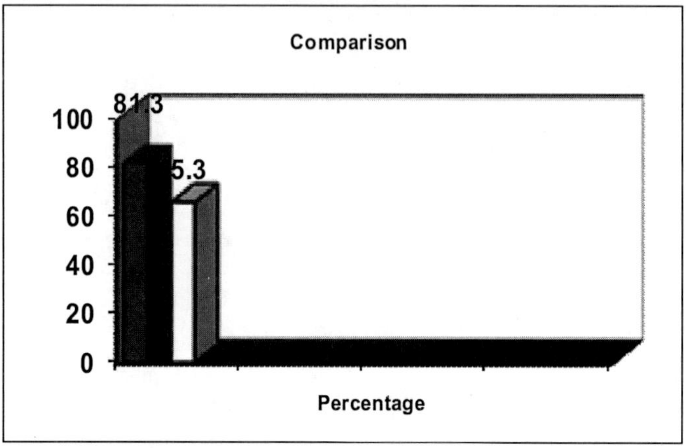

Just like the number of televisions is more both in rural and urban areas, maximum information is obtained about HIV/AIDS from programmes in television. Nearly 81.3% people of the urban areas and 65.3% people of the rural areas agree to this. This is a good trend because providing lot of information will control the spread of this disease.

15. Which is your Favorite Programme?

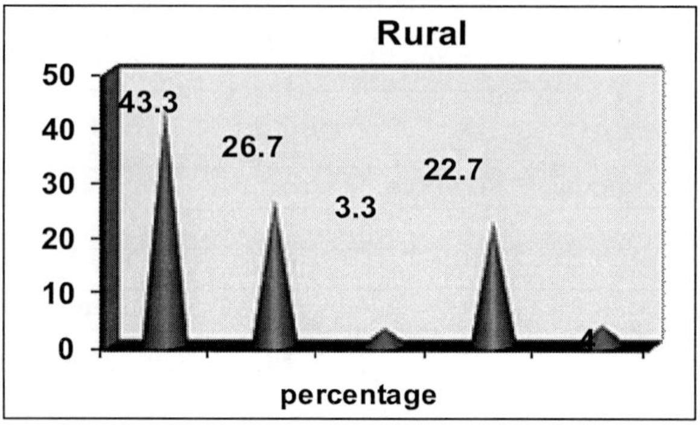

Table No: 15

Description	Respondent	Percentage
Serials	65	43.3
Advertisement	40	26.7
Sports	5	3.3
Health related	34	22.7
Any other	6	4.0
Total	**150**	**100**

43.3% of people responded serials as their favorite programme, 26.7% of people said advertisement as their favorite programme, 22.7% of people said health related programme as their favorite one, 4% of people gave their opinion other than the above said and only 3,3% of people responded sports as their favorite programme.

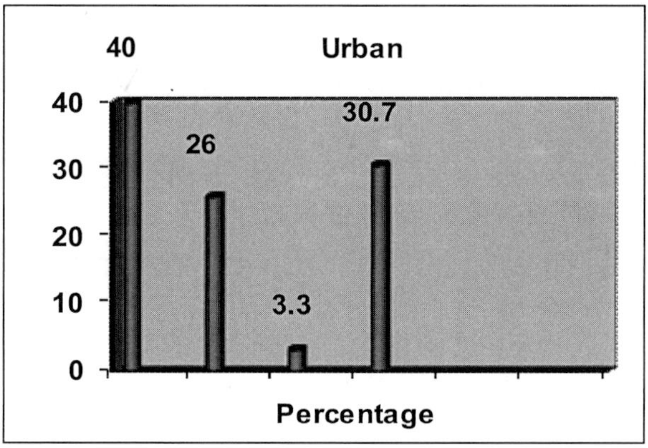

Description	Respondent	Percentage
Serials	60	40.0
Advertisement	39	26.0
Sports	5	3.3
Health related	46	30.7
Total	150	100

The most favorite programme for 40% of the people are serials, for 30.7% of the people it is health related programme, for 26% of it is advertisement, and only 3.3% of the people felt that sports is their favorite programme.

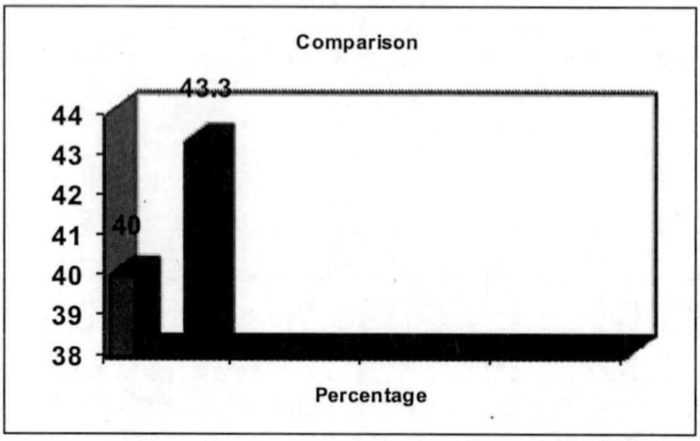

Serials in the television have captured the attention of the viewers both in rural and urban areas. The percentage nearly the same. Rural 43.3% and urban 40%. This shows that entertainment is the chief aim of people. Hence the information about HIV/AIDS can be spread especially through the serials.

16. Do you get Enough Information about HIV/AIDS through media?

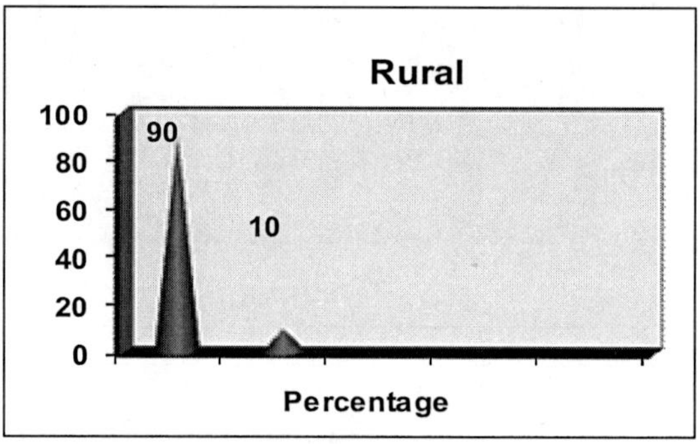

Table No: 16

Description	Respondent	Percentage
Yes	135	90.0
No	15	10.0
Total	**150**	**100**

90% of people answered that they get more information about HIV/AIDS through media and only 10% of people say that they don't get sufficient information through media.

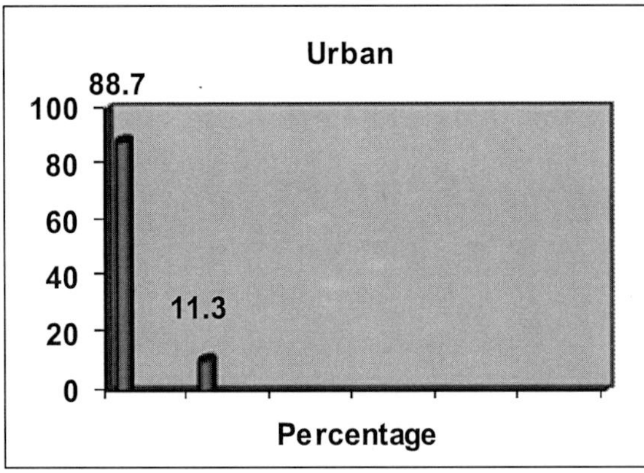

Description	Respondent	Percentage
Yes	133	88.7
No	17	11.3
Total	**150**	**100**

88.7% of people agree that they get enough information about HIV/AIDS through media, and 11.35 of the people say that they don't get sufficient information about HIV/AIDS through media.

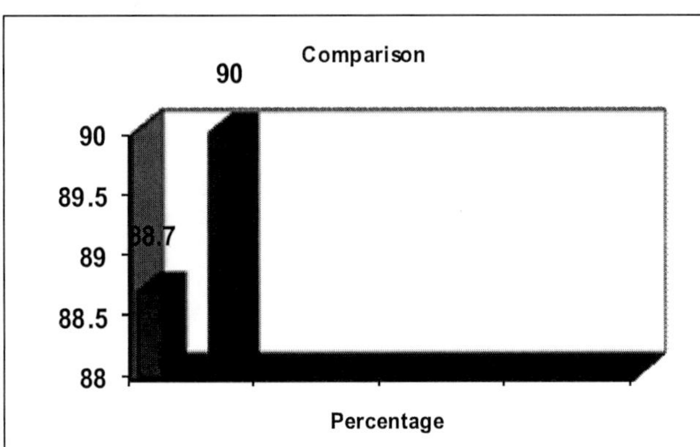

People are appreciative of the media about its part in providing information about HIV/AIDS. Nearly 90% of the rural area population and 88.7% of the urban area population strongly opine that media does a good job in providing enough information. Since this is a dreadful disease more information can be given about the harmful effects.

17. Do you think Media are Powerful to bring Social Awareness in Tamil Nadu on HIV/AIDS?

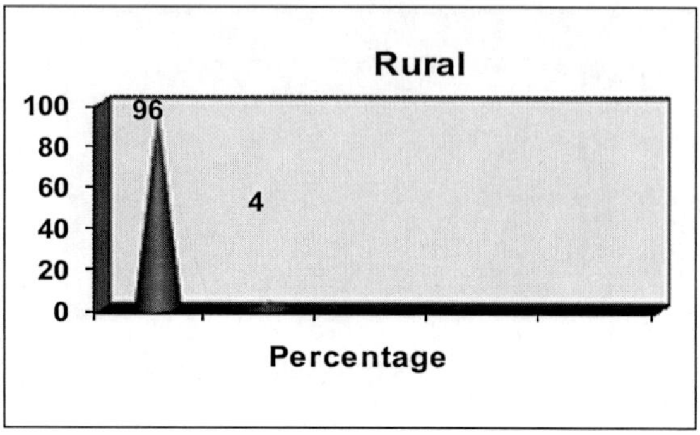

Table No: 17

Description	Respondent	Percentage
Yes	144	96.0
No	6	4.0
Total	**150**	**100**

96% of people feel that media is the powerful weapon to bring social awareness in Tamil Nadu on HIV/AIDS, and only 4% feel that media is not a powerful means to create awareness among people.

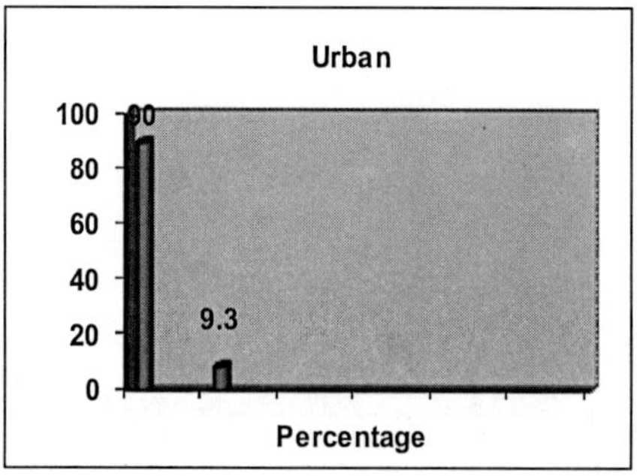

Description	Respondent	Percentage
Yes	136	90.7
No	14	9.3
Total	**150**	**100**

A large number of 90.7% of people felt that media is strong enough to bring social awareness in Tamil Nadu on HIV/AIDS, while only 9.3% of people felt that media is not the powerful one to bring so in Tamil Nadu on the topic HIV/AIDS.

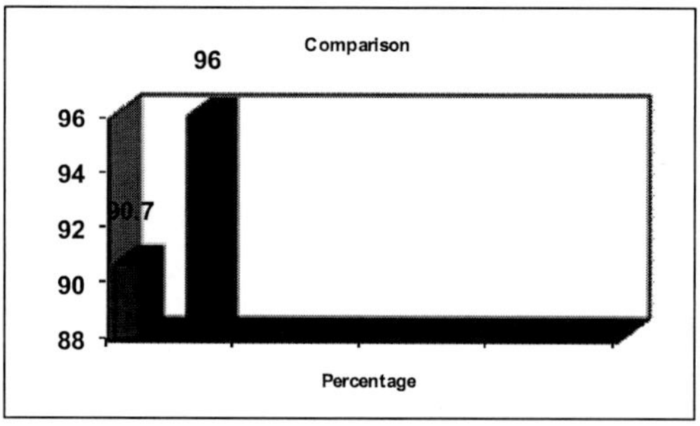

The opinion of the rural and urban population is nearly the same in expressing the idea that media are powerful to bring social awareness in Tamil Nadu on HIV/AIDS. 96% of the rural population and 90.7% of the urban population strongly believe that this can be efficiently done by the media.

Social awareness is an area where something is lacking on the part of the media. The media should focus on this aspect further.

18. Any Latest Cinema or TV Programme, you have seen on HIV?

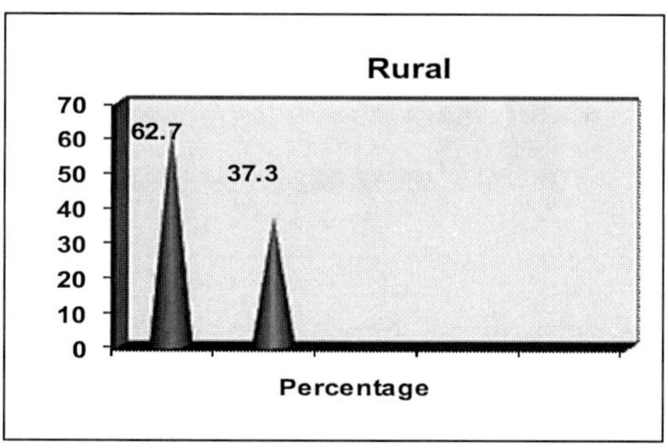

Table No: 18

Description	Respondent	Percentage
Yes	94	62.7
No	56	37.3
Total	**150**	**100**

62.7% of people answered that they have seen cinema and TV programme on the topic of HIV/AIDS, and 37.3% of people said that they have not seen or heard anything about HIV/AIDS from above said media.

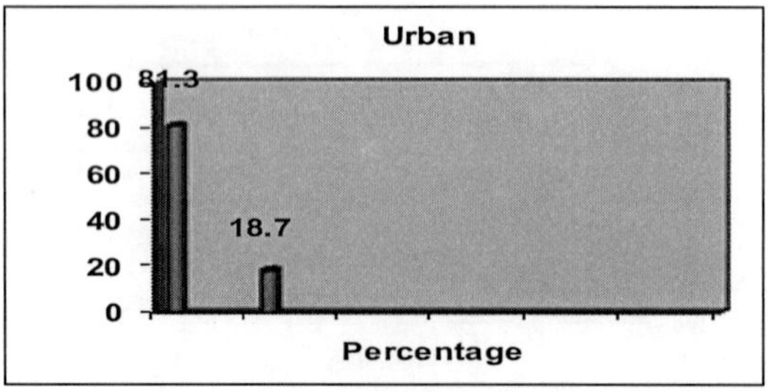

Description	Respondent	Percentage
Yes	122	81.3
No	28	18.7
Total	**150**	**100**

81.3% of people have seen latest cinema or TV programme on HIV, and 18.7% of the people said that they have not seen any latest cinema or TV programme on HIV.

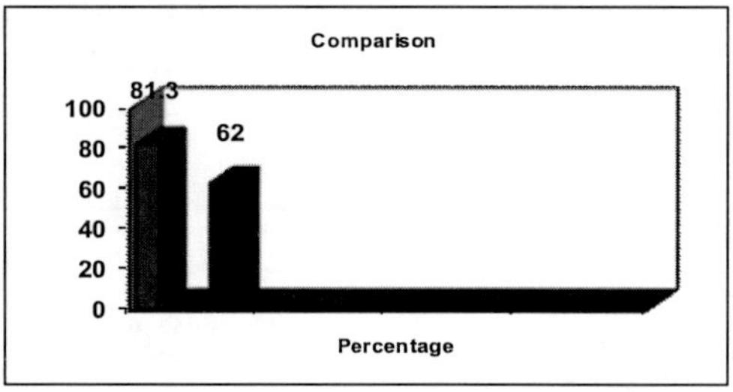

As the government wants to spread the awareness about HIV/AIDS it encourages many agencies to produce serials or even cinemas to create this awareness among the public. Since the events are very interesting both rural and urban people view them. Since cinema is an effective medium in teaching people more films based on this subject can be produced and released.

Positive Attitude towards Hiv/Aids Patient

AIDS and the threat it poses to the stability of communities is one of the focus of this study. AIDS affects the most productive members of society which can lead to the breakdown of family, community and political structures. Widespread and deeply rooted myths about HIV continue to fuel stigma and discrimination against people living with HIV. Media can help bring awareness on this aspect by large scale campaign to promote solidarity with people living with HIV. Civil and international conflicts de scandalise and displace populations increasing vulnerability to HIV infection. What we need to do is to cultivate a positive attitude towards the victims of this virus. Sympathy and moral support to the victims will help them to cope with the situation. One needs to be helped to get out of the paralysis of despair to the ray of hope in life.

The researcher has spent a lot of time to find the aspect of positive support to the victims of HIV/AIDS in this study and see how media can help salvage the situation from despair to hope.

19. I strongly feel that Media can Play a Significant Role to bring out the Right attitude on HIV Patients.

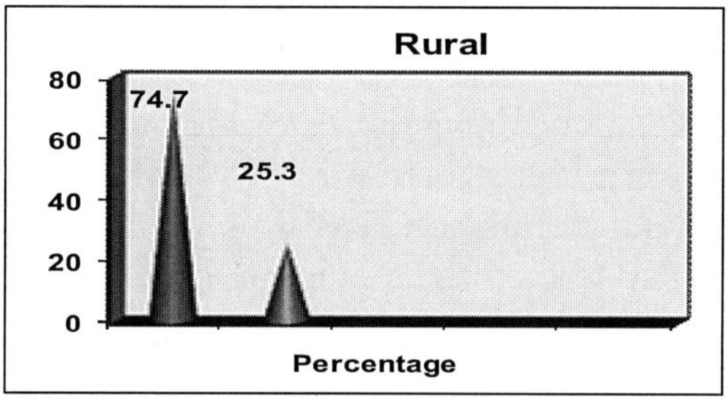

Table No: 19

Description	Respondent	Percentage
Yes	112	74.7
No	38	25.3
Total	**150**	**100**

74.7% of people strongly felt that media can play a significant role to bring out the right attitude on HIV patients and 25.3% of people feel that media doesn't play a significant role to bring out the right attitude on HIV patients.

The majority of the people strongly felt that the media is the only medium which can bring significant role and the right attitude on HIV patients.

Description	Respondent	Percentage
Yes	144	96.0
no	6	4.0
Total	**150**	**100**

A good number of 96% of the propel firmly affirm that media can play a significant role to bring out the right attitude on HIV patients, and only 4% of the people disagreed with the media that plays a significant role to bring out the right attitude on HIV patients.

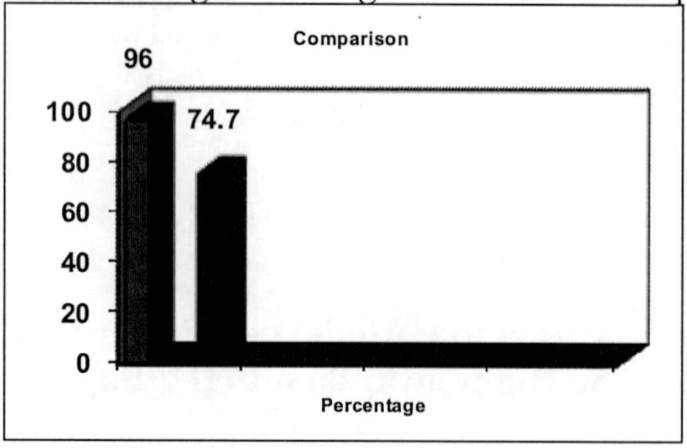

Everyone strongly feels that media can play a significant role among the public in creating a right attitude on HIV patients. This we can understand from the statistics that 96% of urban population and 74.7% of the rural population have this opinion. This opinion is a reasonable one and role of the media can never be exaggerated.

20. I Learnt from Media that Eating with HIV/AIDS Patients is not Harmful.

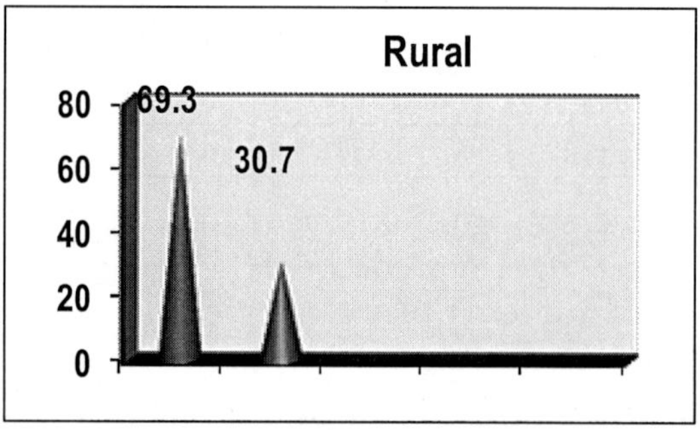

Table No: 20

Description	Respondent	Percentage
Yes	104	69.3
No	46	30.7
Total	**150**	**100**

69.3% of people learnt from media that eating with HIV/AIDS patients is not harmful, and on the other hand 30.7% of people feel that they learnt from media that eating with HIV/AIDS patients is harmful.

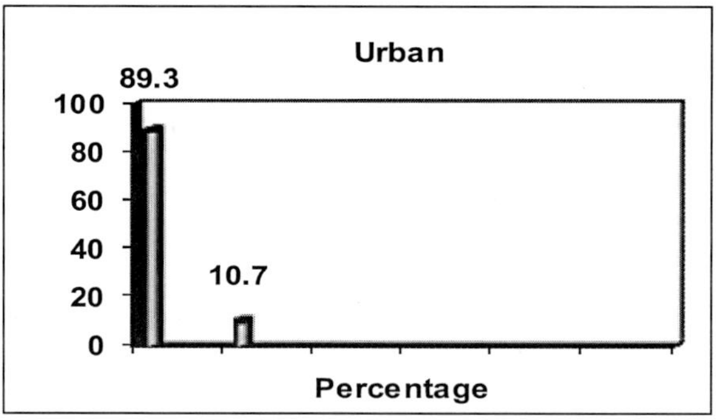

Description	Respondent	Percentage
Yes	134	89.3
no	16	10.7
Total	**150**	**100**

89.3% of the people learnt from media that eating with HIV/AIDS patients is not harmful, and 10.7% of the people oppose the above response and said that it is harmful to eat with the HIV/AIDS patients.

It is good to know that media has taught the people positively while dealing with the HIV/AIDS patient.

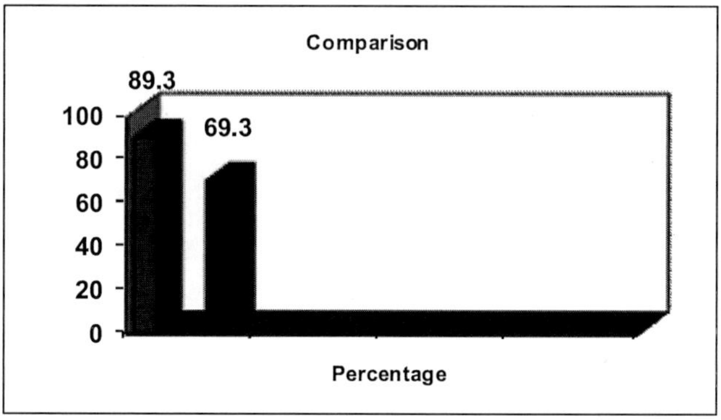

It is happy to note that many consider that sitting and eating with the HIV affected persons is not harmful. 89.3% of the urban population and 69.3% of the rural population believed this. Here also we can notice from the urban and rural percentages that this belief is less in village areas. Due to ignorance villagers think even sitting with them may spread the disease. This false belief can be nullified by the media.

21. Media Taught me that I can Exchange my Dress and other Materials with the HIV/AIDS Patients without being affected.

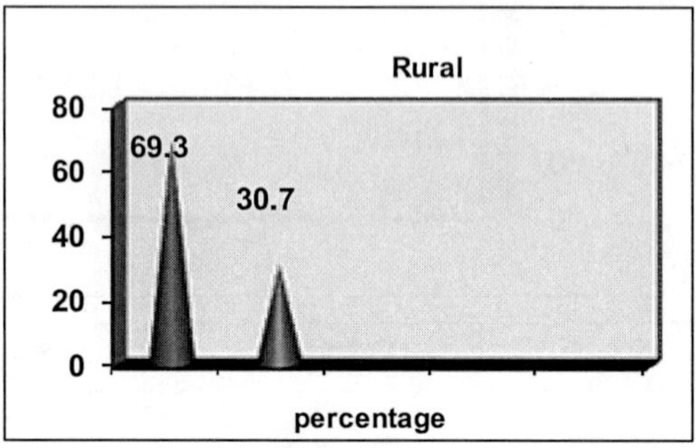

Table No: 21

Description	Respondent	Percentage
Yes	100	66.7
No	50	33.3
Total	**150**	**100**

66.7% of people agree that media taught them that they can exchange their dress and other materials with the HIV/AIDS patients without being affected, whereas 33.3% of people disagree with the above point.

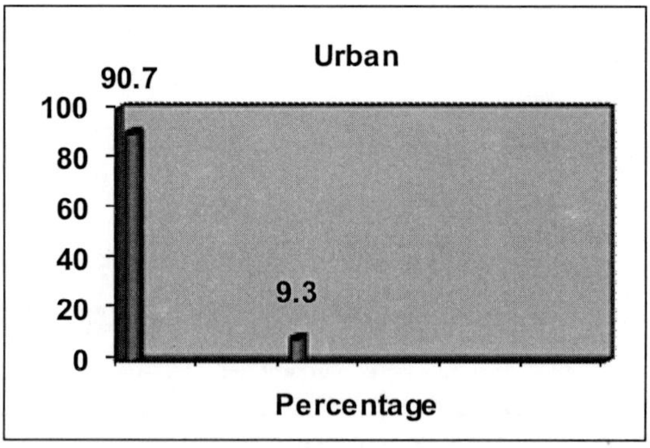

Description	Respondent	Percentage
Yes	136	90.7
no	14	9.3
Total	**150**	**100**

Media taught to 90.7% of the people that they can exchange their dress and other materials with the HIV/AIDS patients without being affected, and 9.3% of the people just deny the above affirmed statement.

It is significant to note that media plays a great role in providing right views in dealing with the HIV/AIDS affected patients.

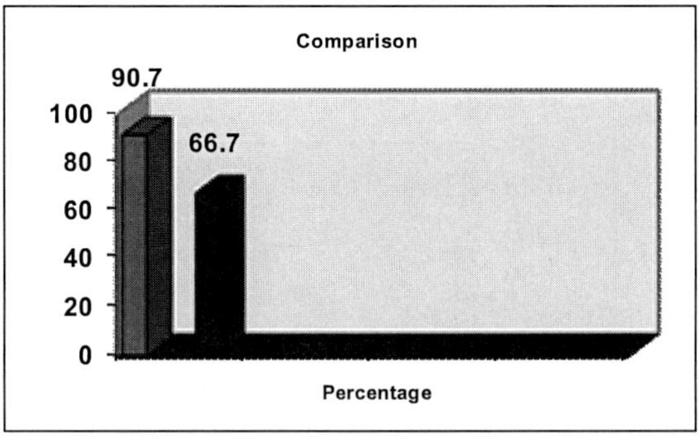

People had a wrong notion that if we exchange our clothing or other materials with the HIV patients we will be affected. The media dispelled this wrong notion from the public. Now nearly 90.7% of urban people and 66.7% of the rural people don't believe the above fallacy. Here again we note that village folk are still a bit hesitant. Lack of knowledge about this disease is the main reason. This can be reduced slowly by the media with its propaganda.

22. TV, Radio, Magazines and News Papers on HIV/AIDS have helped me to Change my Attitude towards the people affected by HIV/AIDS.

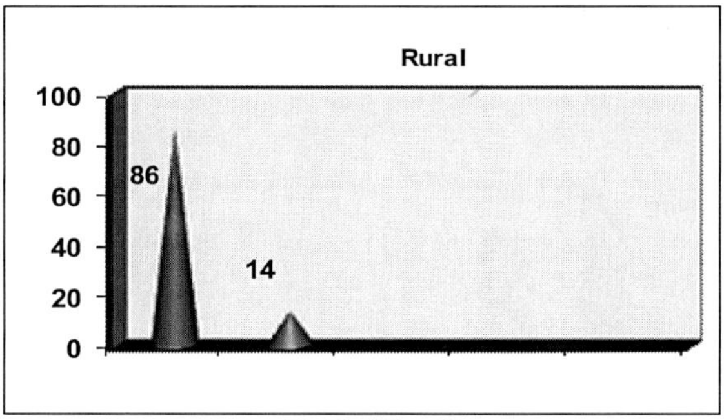

Table No: 22

Description	Respondent	Percentage
Yes	129	86.0
No	21	14.0
Total	**150**	**100**

86% of people say that TV, radio, magazines and newspapers on HIV/AIDS have helped them to change their attitude towards the people affected by HIV/AIDS, but 14% of people say that the above said medium is not helping them to change their attitude towards the people affected by HIV/AIDS.

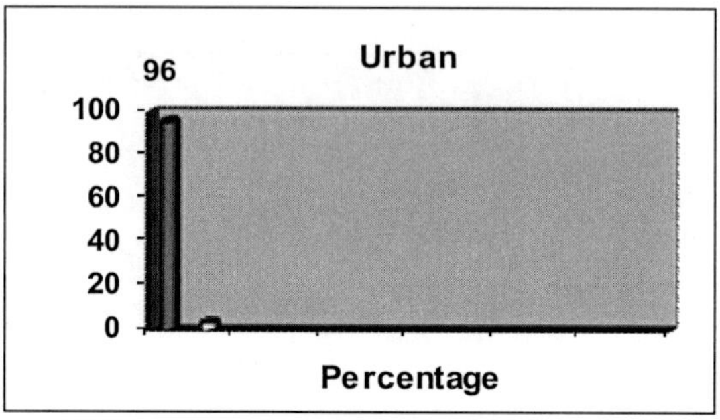

Description	Respondent	Percentage
Yes	144	96.0
no	6	4.0
Total	**150**	**100**

For the above question a great number of 96% of people responded that the media such as, TV, radio, magazines and newspapers on HIV/AIDS have helped them to change their attitude towards the people affected by HIV/AIDS, but on the other hand only 4% of the people deny that TV, radio, magazines and newspapers on HIV/AIDS have helped them to change their attitude towards the people affected by HIV/AIDS.

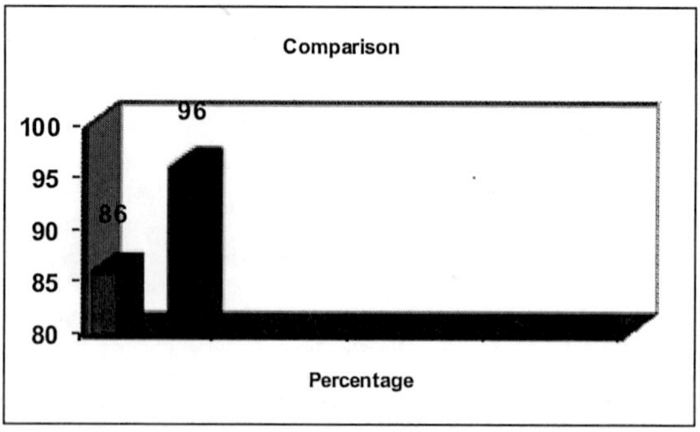

It is really commendable that the media like TV and radio have played a very significant role in changing the attitude of the people towards the HIV/AIDS patients. Media has played a more important role in the rural areas 96% than in the urban areas 86%.

23. My Attitude towards the HIV/AIDS Affected Patients has Changed due to Media Information

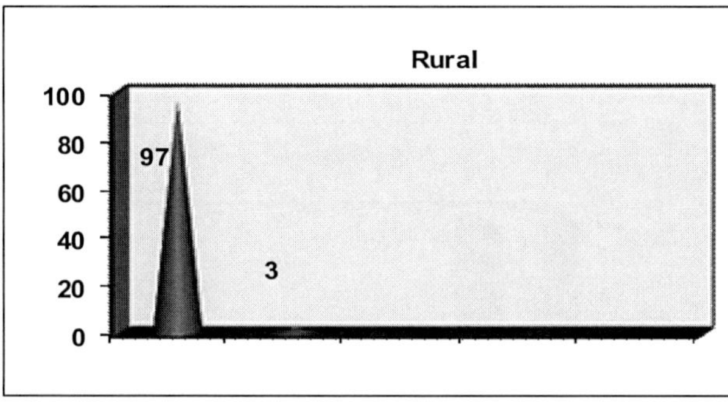

Table No: 23

Description	Respondent	Percentage
Yes	145	97
No	5	3
Total	**150**	**100**

96.7% of people's attitude towards the HIV/AIDS affected patients have changed to media information, while only 3.3% of people are not convinced that their attitude towards the HIV/AIDS affected patients did not change due to media information.

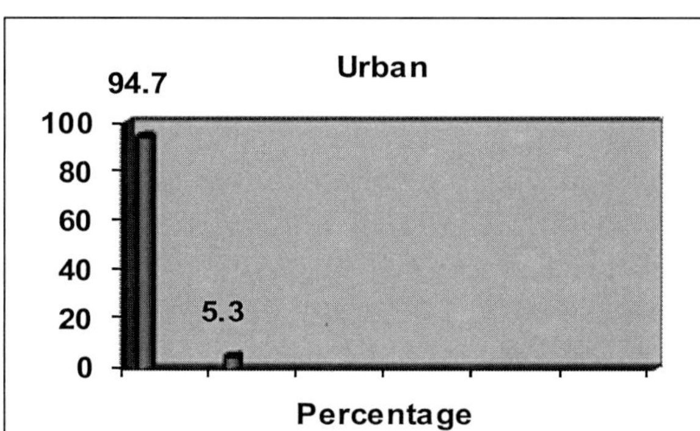

Description	Respondent	Percentage
Yes	142	94.7
No	8	5.3
Total	**150**	**100**

It was responded by 94.7% of the people that they changed their attitude towards the HIV/AIDS affected patients due to the media information, but only 5.3% of the people did not have any change in their attitude towards the HIV/AIDS affected patients due to the media information.

It is very pleasing to note that media changed positively the attitudes of many people towards the HIV/AIDS affected patients.

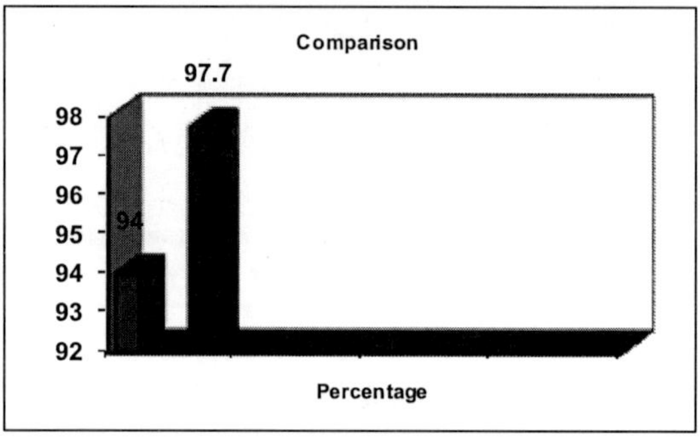

Nearly 94.7% of the urban population and 97.7% of the rural population have issued strong statements that only due to media information they have changed their attitude towards the HIV/AIDS patients. Only a minimum percentage of people have not changed and in due course media will attain that achievement also. This is a very good trend for socialization for the up liftmen of the society.

Media Methods of Prevention

Across the world, a small but growing number of countries have reduced HIV/AIDS prevalence through sound prevention efforts. However, in 2005 there were still 4.1 million new adult infections occurring among young people aged 15-25. According to latest estimates, HIV prevention services reach only one in ten of those most at risk. (UNAIDS REPORT – 14, August, 2006) in an era where the world has committed to work towards universal access to HIV prevention, treatment, care and support, there is clearly an urgent need to intensify HIV prevention efforts in both size and scale to halt growing infection rates and sustain the gains that have already been made in the AIDS RESPONSE SUCH AS INCREASED NUMBERS OF people on HIV treatment. In this connection the media can bring pressure on the village or town groups to priorities HIV PREVENTION

These studies will bring out such measures as much as possible by the research.

24. Do you know HIV/AIDS can be prevented through media?

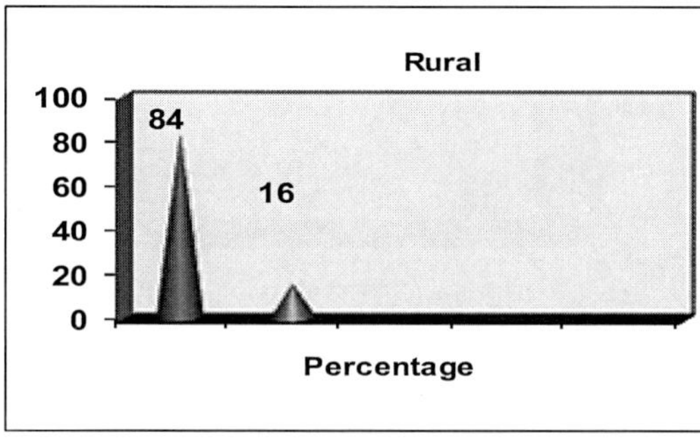

Table No: 24

Description	Respondent	Percentage
Yes	126	84.0
No	24	16.0
Total	**150**	**100**

84% of people affirm that HIV/AIDS can be prevented through media, whereas 16% of people deny that HIV/AIDS can be prevented through media.

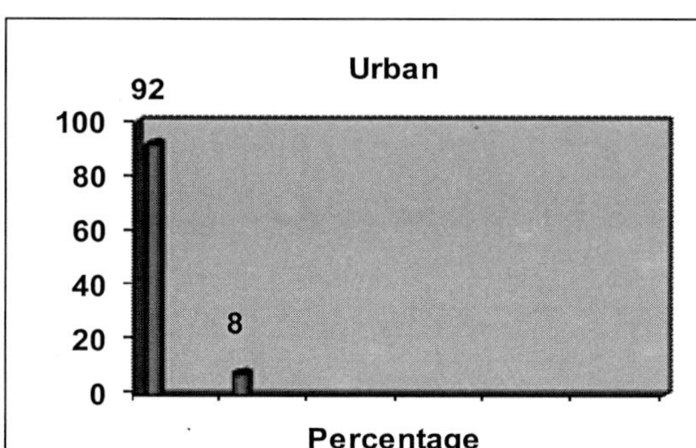

Description	Respondent	Percentage
Yes	138	92.0
no	12	8.0
Total	**150**	**100**

92% of people knew that HIV/AIDS can be prevented through media and only 8% of the people did not know that HIV/AIDS can be prevented through media.

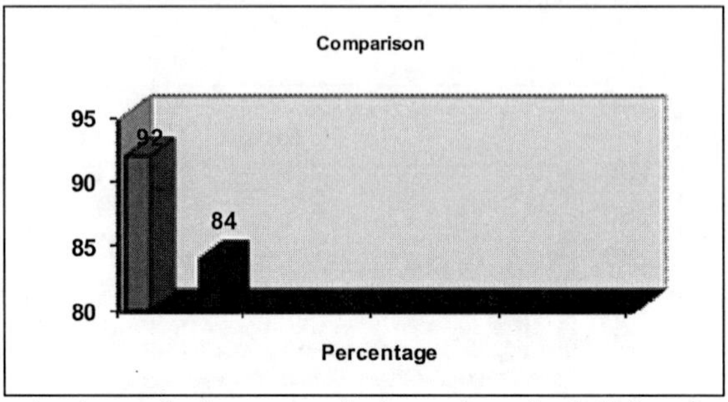

A vast majority of the population that is 84% of the rural and 92% of the urban, very strongly believe that HIV/AIDS can be prevented through media only. This shows us the importance of media in preventing the same. We have already stressed in many places about the importance of media in preventing the disease.

25. Have you ever come across any Programme in TV or Radio on HIV/AIDS Prevention Method?

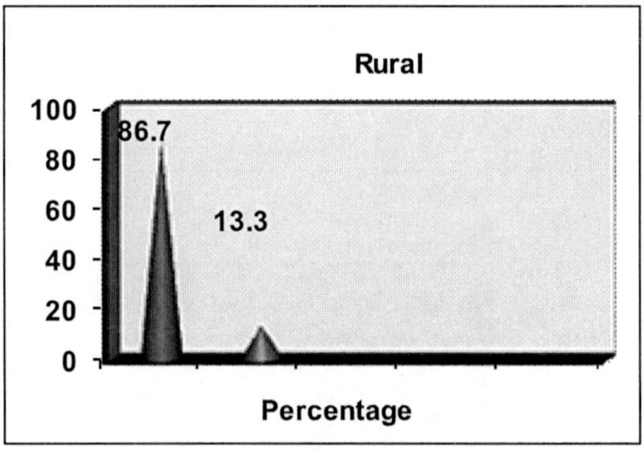

Table No: 25

Description	Respondent	Percentage
Yes	130	86.7
No	20	13.3
Total	**150**	**100**

86.7% of people say that they have come across porgrammes in TV and radio on HIV/AIDS prevention method, but 13.3% people have never come across such programmes on HIV/AIDS prevention method.

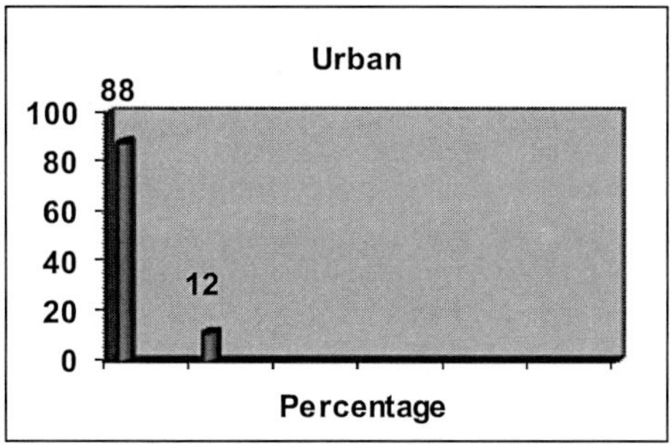

Description	Respondent	Percentage
Yes	132	88.0
no	18	12.0
Total	**150**	**100**

For the above mentioned question 88% of people had come across few programmes on TV and Radio on HIV/AIDS prevention, where as 12% of the people said that they had never come across any programme in TV or Radio of HIV/AIDS prevention.

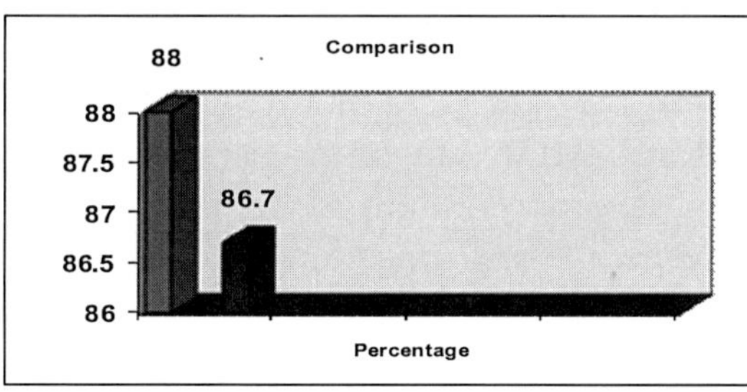

Many people, 88% from the urban area and 86.7% from the rural area have come across programmes about the prevention of HIV/AIDS and it has strengthened their conviction that HIV/AIDS can be prevented. This shows that we are traveling in the right direction and a day may come that "prevention "may become the keyword.

26. How can you Prevent getting AIDS?

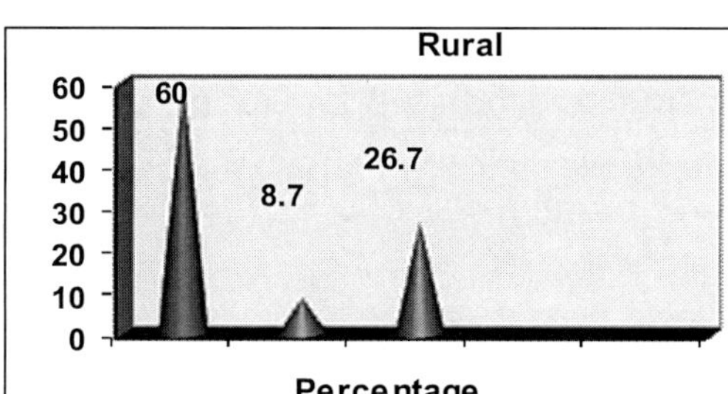

AIDS can be prevented through various ways, according to 60% of people AIDS can be prevented through protected sex, 26.7% of people suggested proper use of condom, 8.7% of people say through faithful partner, and 4.7% of people say that they do not know.

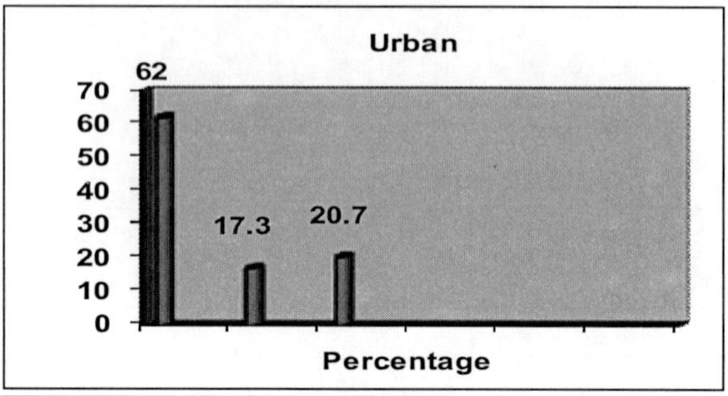

Description	Respondent	Percentage
Protected sex	93	62.0
Faithful partner	26	17.3
Use condom	31	20.7
Total	**150**	**100**

Many responses had come from different people for how to prevent getting AIDS. They are: 62% of the people answered that by practicing protected sex AIDS can be prevented, 20.7% of people felt that the proper usage of condom is the way to prevent getting AIDS, 17.3% of the people said that the best preventive method is none other than having faithful partner.

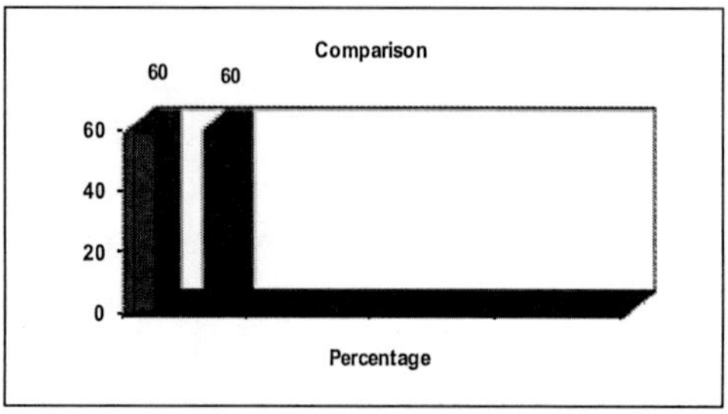

The major portion of the population is of the view that only by following protected sex people can prevent getting AIDS. Nearly 60% of both the rural and urban population very strongly believe in this theory. The most important aspect of the disease is the preventive one and "protected sex" is the key word in preventing this disease.

27. Has any Medium helped you to know about Prevention Methods?

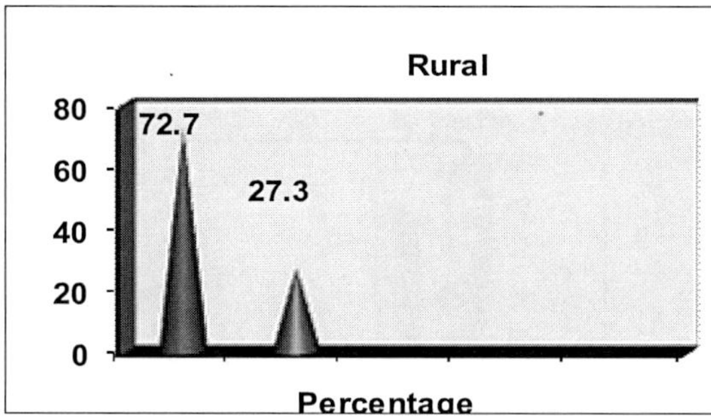

Table No: 27

Description	Respondent	Percentage
Yes	109	72.7
No	41	27.3
Total	**150**	**100**

72.7% of people were helped by media to know about prevention methods, and 27.3% of people say that they were not helped by media to know about the prevention methods.

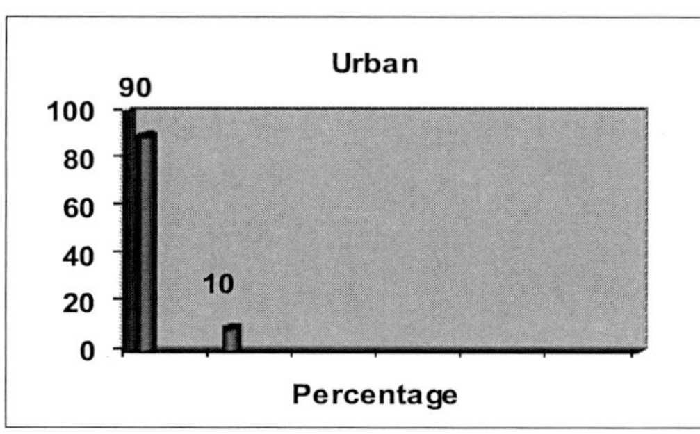

Description	Respondent	Percentage
Yes	135	90.0
no	15	10.0
Total	**150**	**100**

90% of people say that they were helped by media to know about prevention methods, and 10% of the people concretely said that none of the medium helped them to know about prevention methods.

From the above table we are certain that media plays a vital role for the welfare of the society, particularly to have a proper preventive method of HIV/AIDS.

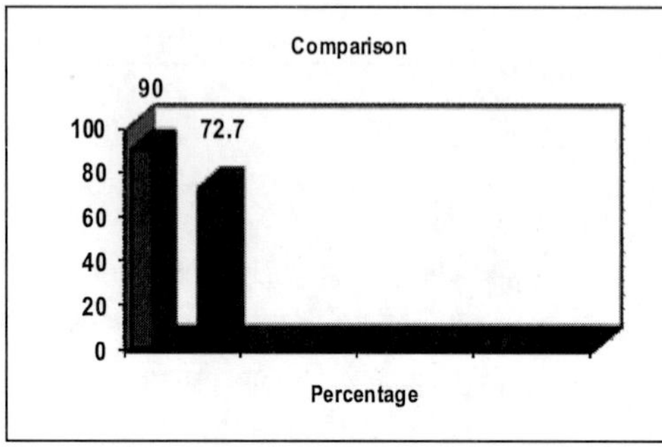

90% of the urban population emphatically states that the preventive methods were taught to them by the media alone. Though less, 72.7% rural population also subscribes to this concept. Here the importance of the media is stressed.

28. Have you Heard from the Media the usage of Condom?

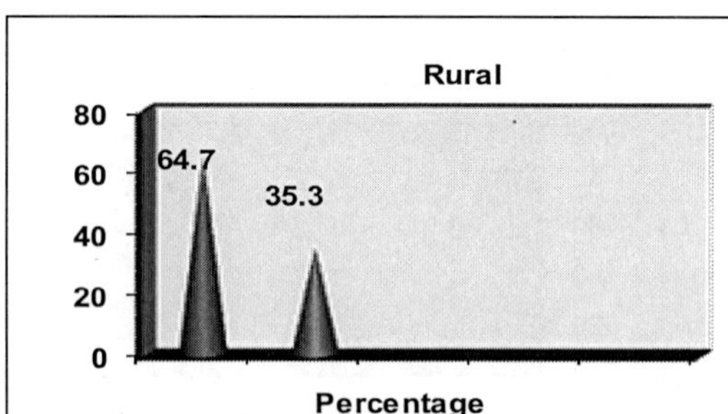

Table No: 28

Description	Respondent	Percentage
Yes	97	64.7
No	53	35.3
Total	**150**	**100**

64.7% of people have heard from the media the usage of condom and 35.3% of people have not heard from the media the usage of condom.

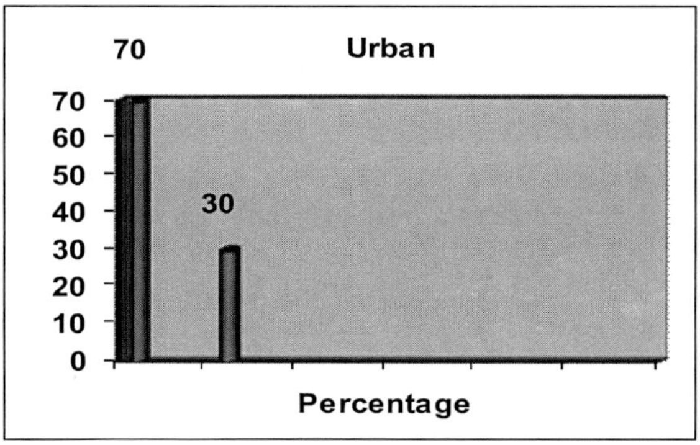

Description	Respondent	Percentage
Yes	105	70.0
no	45	30.0
Total	**150**	**100**

70% of the people had heard from the media the proper usage of condom, and 30% of the people say that they did not hear form the media the right usage of condom.

Here it is very important to note that a good number of 70% of people came to the awareness of the proper use of condom from the media.

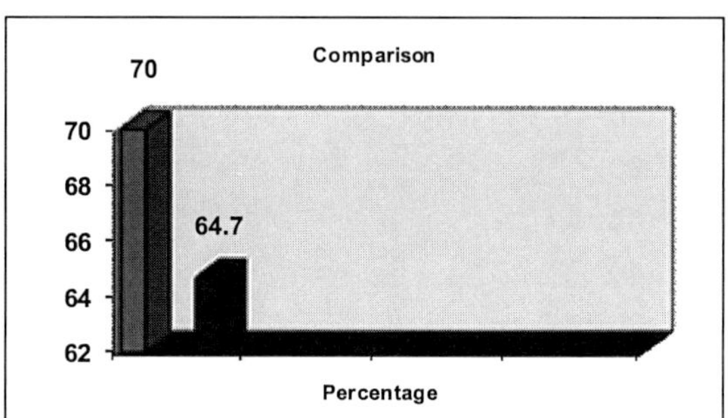

Usage of condom is considered to be an important step in safe sex and 70% of the urban population and 64.7% rural population know about its usage. Prevention goes in the right direction. The government can teach the importance of using condoms through the media.

29. Do you think Media can help Safe Blood Transfusion to Stop spread of HIV/AIDS?

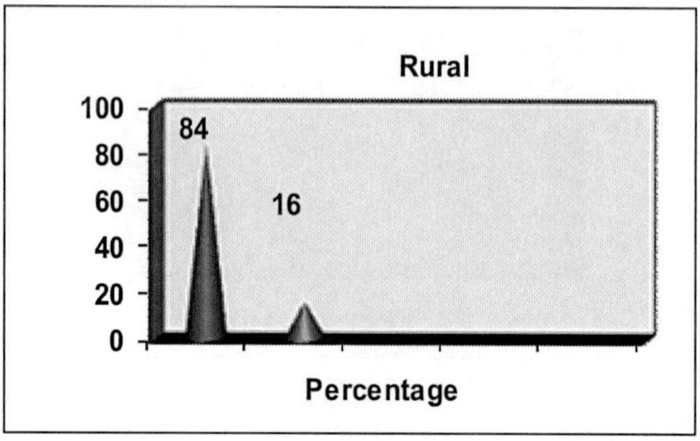

Table No: 29

Description	Respondent	Percentage
Yes	126	84.0
No	24	16.0
Total	**150**	**100**

84% of people feel that media can help safe blood transfusion to stop spread of HIV/AIDS, on the other side 16% of the people oppose that the media can help safe blood transfusion to stop spread of HIV/AIDS.

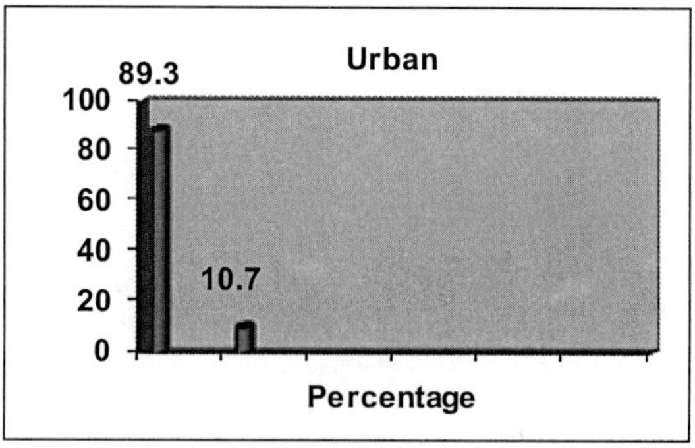

Description	Respondent	Percentage
Yes	134	89.3
no	16	10.7
Total	**150**	**100**

89.3% of the people said with firm confidence that media is so powerful that can help safe blood transfusion to stop spread of

HIV/AIDS, while 10.7% of the people suggested that media can't help safe blood transfusion to stop spread of HIV/AIDS.

From the above table it is vividly clear that the effect of the media to help the people to have the clear knowledge about even the safe blood transfusion to stop spread of HIV/AIDS.

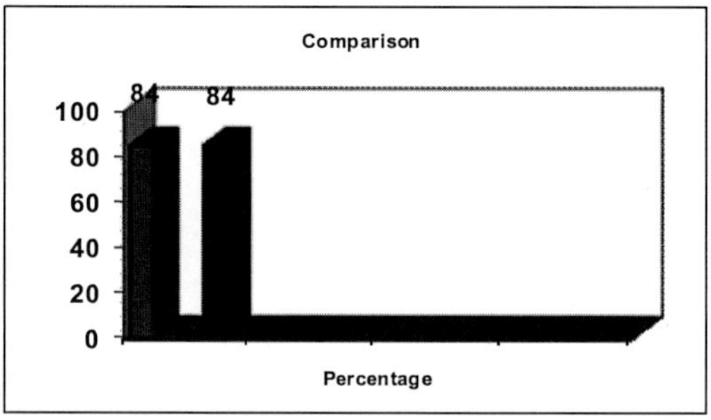

Blood transfusion is thought to be one of the causes for the spreading HIV/AIDS and people very strongly believe that media can play a very important role in educating the people about safe transfusion of blood. On an average nearly 84% of the people both rural and urban believe this and they say that media only educated them. Blood transfusion has become a necessity due to various medical reasons and sometimes this causes AIDS. Hence safe transfusion of blood should be given importance by the people of the medical profession.

30. Do you think Media can Educate on Safe Sex to stop Spread of HIV/AIDS?

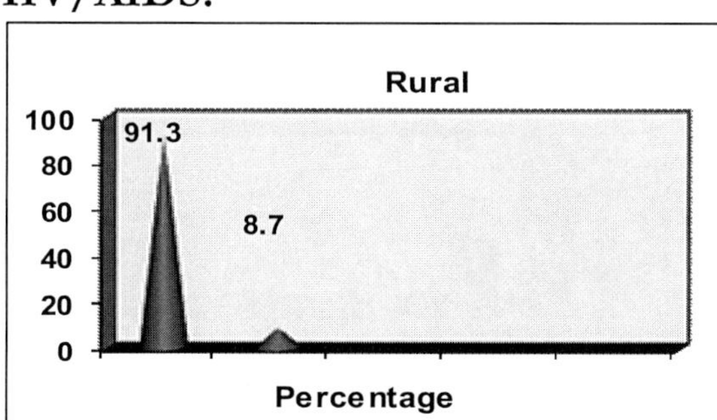

Table No: 30

Description	Respondent	Percentage
Yes	137	91.3
No	13	8.7
Total	**150**	**100**

91.3% of people agree with the media that it can be a helpful means to educate on safe sex to stop spread of **HIV/AIDS,** while 8.7% of people say that media can't be helpful to educate on safe sex to stop spread of **HIV/AIDS**.

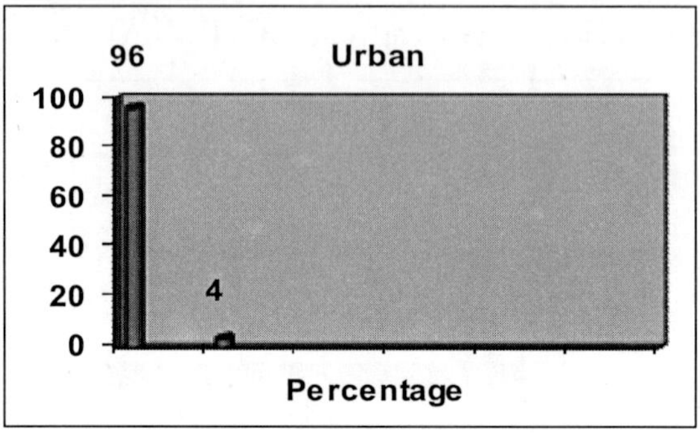

Description	Respondent	Percentage
Yes	144	96.0
no	6	4.0
Total	**150**	**100**

For the above question 96% of people felt that media can play the role of a good educator on safe sex to stop spread of HIV/AIDS, and only 4% of the people said that media can't be in any way possible to be the educator on safe sex to stop spread of HIV/AIDS.

Once again from the above table we are clear enough about the positive effect of media of safe sex to stop spread of HIV/AIDS.

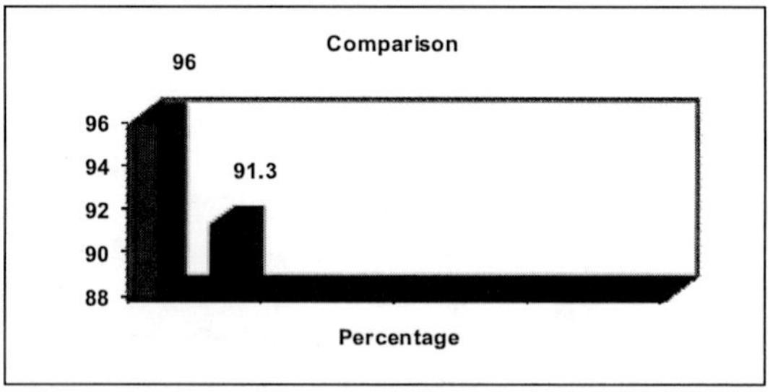

The knowledge spread by the media about safe sex is an authoritative one. Safe sex is one of the important preventive measures. 96% of the urban population and 91.3% of rural population have high hopes about the media in this service. Let this aspect be given wide publicity and the people be saved from the curse of this disease.

CHAPTER 5

Findings and Suggestions

- People whether they are from villages or towns know that HIV/ AIDS is a killer disease. So far only cancer was considered as the most dreadful disease but now people have understood that HIV/ AIDS is worse than that.
- A very low percentage of people still think that AIDS spreads even if clothes are exchanged or when a person sits and eats with an AIDS patient. Many know that the disease is spread only through sexual contact. Though scientific many know that the disease is caused by virus.
- Many people who contact AIDS do not know the symptoms. But of late through the media, people have started understanding through symptoms like lack of appetite, loss of weight and physical weakness.
- Many people think that if a person gets AIDS his tenure of life will be only five or ten years. Many do not know that new medicines have been produced and they can prolong life upto30 years.
- One unfortunate thing is if a mother who is pregnant has AIDS the child also catches AIDS. Some know that Navarapin can be used to prevent this spread of disease from the mother to the child.
- All agencies which work for the prevention of this disease pay more attention to the preventive aspect of this disease than for the curative aspect.
- Though information is available about this killer disease, media like TV and radio pay a major role in spreading the message. Especially TV and cinema which are very attractive media catch the attention of the people very easily. Moreover these messages reach millions of people at a time and people are kept informed about all the aspects of this killer disease.

Films and serials are produced using this theme and people view it with interest.

- Many people have categorically stated in the questionnaire that they have gathered maximum information only from the media like radio, TV and cinema.
- Media, cinema, T.V make many to lose their control and seek sex which was one of the causes of HIV/AIDS spread.
- Most women talked freely and gave general opinion on consolidated problem, feelings, and sufferings of other people. People in city were a bit hesitant to talk openly on HIV related matters, whereas, the rural folk was very spontaneous.
- It was observed that most of the women take a lot of pride of being educated. Rural women long for education and are happy to say that "I have studied up to 5th Standard" shows they have love for education and media attraction.
- The main theme, the media concentrate is creating a social awareness among the public about this killer disease. Unfortunately either due to ignorance or due to some stigma the AIDS affected people are looked down by others or to some extent it creates a social segregation. The patients suffer more mentally than physiologically and may lead to quicker death. This noble work of creating social awareness is done by the media.
- Now because of the media propaganda, public are aware of the facts like causes of the disease, how it spreads, medicines available to mitigate the seriousness of the disease how the patients should be treated by the society and what all steps can be taken to prevent the disease. The main thing that people come to know that protected sex alone can prevent this disease.
- We have already seen that people are very much interested in serials in TV. Hence Governments can subsidies the cost in producing TV serials based on the all effects of the AIDS.
- We have learnt that TV is the most powerful medium in spreading any information and hence the information about AIDS also spreads. Since TV is a bit costly people below poverty line have no easy access to it. Hence government can distribute free TV sets or at subsidized rates. (The

Government of Tamil Nadu has taken up this job and is distributing free TV'S to poor people.)

- From the questionnaire, we could find that use of condoms were not much prevalent among rural men folk. They even feel shy to talk about it. They can be made to come out of that shyness. We understand that in remote villages pregnant women normally don't go for medical checkups not even for general medical checkup. And these women because of ignorance never think about contacted AIDS. This might have spread from the husband and she as faithful women never suspected her husband. This is a tradition being followed by women of our land.

Suggestions

- Awareness and advertisement must be given on Sundays and holidays for half an hour in the T.V. or Radio or so in the form of songs, dramas, or skits or talk by experts on HIV/AIDS. Because many people watch TV on Sunday This will make an impact in the rural and urban areas.
- The Press groups, NGOs, NCC or College groups should reach the problem from grassroots level. As group the Media must net-work to cover a few villages depending on the village populations. They must camp in the village for at least 30 days to provide awareness programmes to women. They should repeat it every three months. This way the media can play a vital role to bring awareness among the women in rural and urban set up.
- Doctors and Media persons must strongly insist the male partner to take HIV test when wife is infected and when husband is infected they must insist test be done for the wives. Media can bring awareness programme in their own areas.
- First of all people should be made to understand that HIV/ AIDS is a killer disease and once contacted death is imminent within a short period.
- The parental responsibility towards the children should be stressed. They should be made to think that if the father dies what will happen to the children and his wife too.

- Unfortunately moral standards have gone down in our country now, due to technological advance. Religion should play a role in moralizing the people especially "one man one wife" theory should be widely propagated.
- Prostitution should be dealt with very strictly by the governments.
- All the media should be activated more to spread the message of "one man one wife"
- Sexual weakness is prevalent among human beings. Hence safe sex or protected sex should be taught to the people through media.
- Pregnancy can be terminated at early stages to prevent the offspring contacting the disease.
- It is unfortunate that people in the lower strata of the society are the most affected by the disease. The agencies should concentrate on this area and constant propaganda should be carried out there.
- Keeping constant propaganda should be carried out there.
- Safer methods of blood transfusion should be adopted to prevent the disease from spreading through blood transfusion
- Social gatherings may be arranged and the HIV/AIDS affected patients and the normal people can be brought together, where it can be explained that simple body contacts like touching the patient shall not cause the disease.
- Condoms help men to have safe sex. Now almost all the villages should be covered in the distribution of condoms and they should be informed about the benefits of the same by men medical social workers. Since the government distributes them freely it can be made to use without fail.

CHAPTER 6

Conclusion

In olden days plague was considered as the most serious disease. Many people died and it changed the course of wars too. But those were the days when the scientific and medical field causes miracles and wonderful medicines have been invented to increase the longevity of man's life. But as a challenge to this medical profession, the HIV/AIDS has cropped up and it has become the concern of the whole world. Medical research is going on in this subject and may be invented to kill this killer disease. But within these few years millions of people may die. Hence only preventive aspect is given importance.

In the book "Identity and Violence – The illusion of Destiny, author Amartya Sen has said that the tendency to take a compartmentalized view of identity is the root cause of many conflicts in today's world. He further asserted that the awareness is the first step to any education either in rural or urban set-up. Perhaps taking a leaf from that, the researcher has ventured into the area of awareness with the use of Mass Media Communications in Rural and Urban areas of Chennai with extra dash of depth. Fully aware of the tall order of this project yet the researcher has come out with a few unique findings. The researcher believes that the findings of this thesis might generate a new movement in creating new roles for the media to penetrate into the lives of many in our country.

Public Awareness on HIV/AIDS through media is the subject studied among the Self Help Groups of Keechalam and Saidapet in Chennai using empirical data by personal interviews. First of all the respondents were interviewed on: Age, Education, Occupation, Income and Family Members. Secondly, over 30 questions were prepared and processed with Frequency Table. Finally, these findings were compared scientifically to bring out the real situation as it is today.

Mass media in general are an important force for influencing public opinion and stimulating debate and creating awareness on HIV/AIDS. HIV infection and women as victims – is reported in the media have stimulated debate ever since the virus was detected in Tamil Nadu. The researcher carried out a study to analyze the level of awareness among the women of rural and urban areas of Chennai. Television is the most preferred media, followed by Radio and Cinema. Major source of information on HIV/AIDS was through T.V, Radio and cinema. Awareness level varies from group to group according to their social and educational background. Majority feels that the government should provide HIV/AIDS related education on a constant basis. One of the main findings is that the media and the Department of Health should further educate the people on HIV/AIDS.

The study enlightened the mind of the researcher that the women both in rural and urban are prone to this disease due to ignorance. Only through proper exercise of awareness this evil can be eradicated from the society. When both husband and wife are properly educated the vulnerability is minimum. Obviously, the media can play a significant role to effect this revolution. Was it not a single experience in South Africa that inspired Mohandoss Gandhi to become a Mahatma who propounded his Satyagraha Movement!

A strange thing that is noticed by all is that in spite of all these steps the percentage of this disease is seen on the increase? Why? Let more research be conducted to find out the causes for this too.

Volunteers of Self-Help-Groups

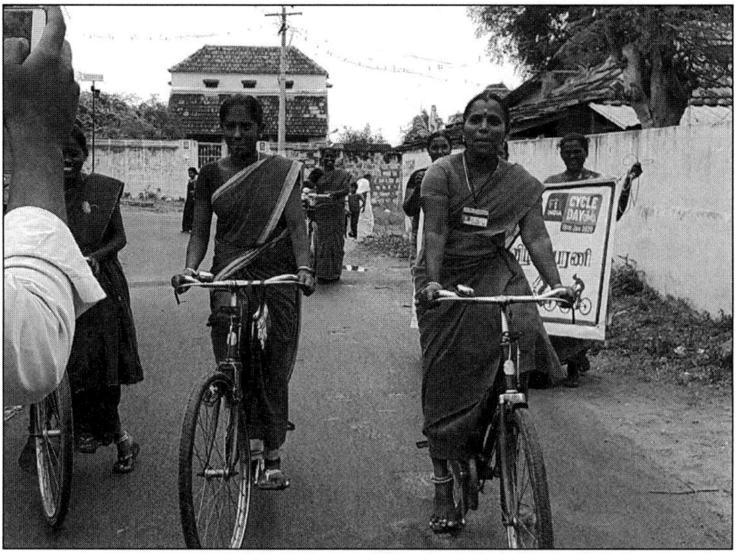

Volunteers peddling to villages

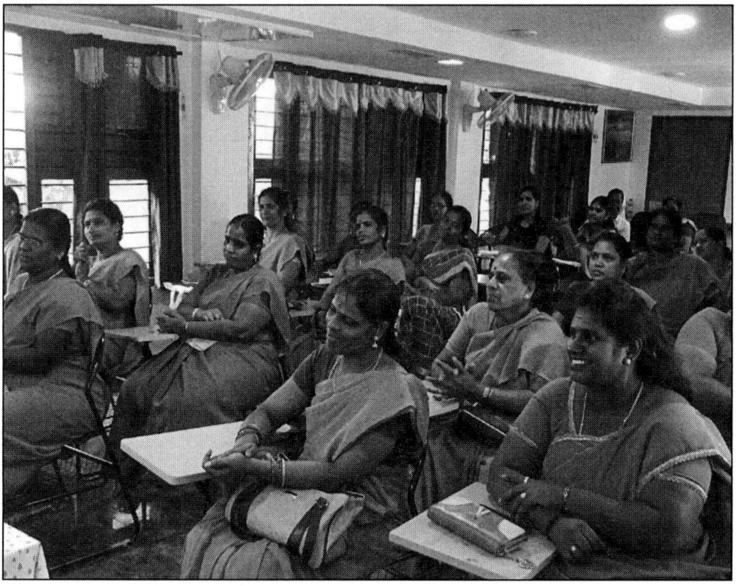

Core-Group Meeting

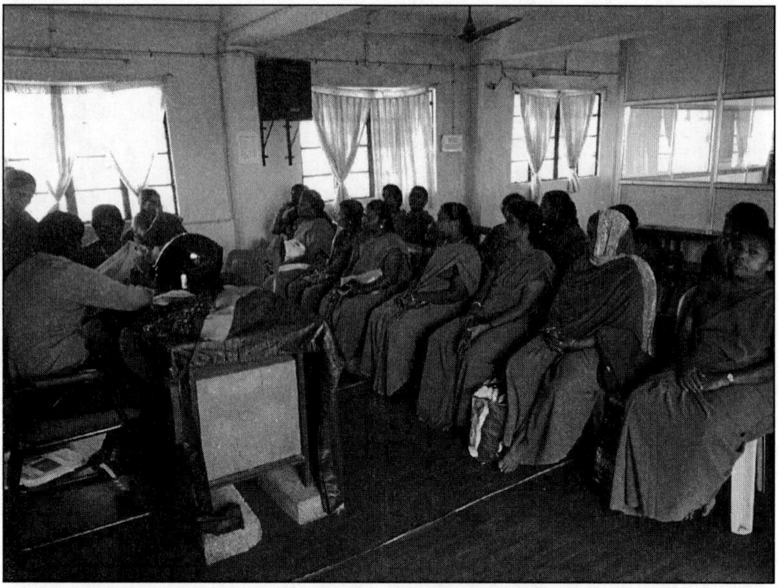

Self-Help-Group with the Patients

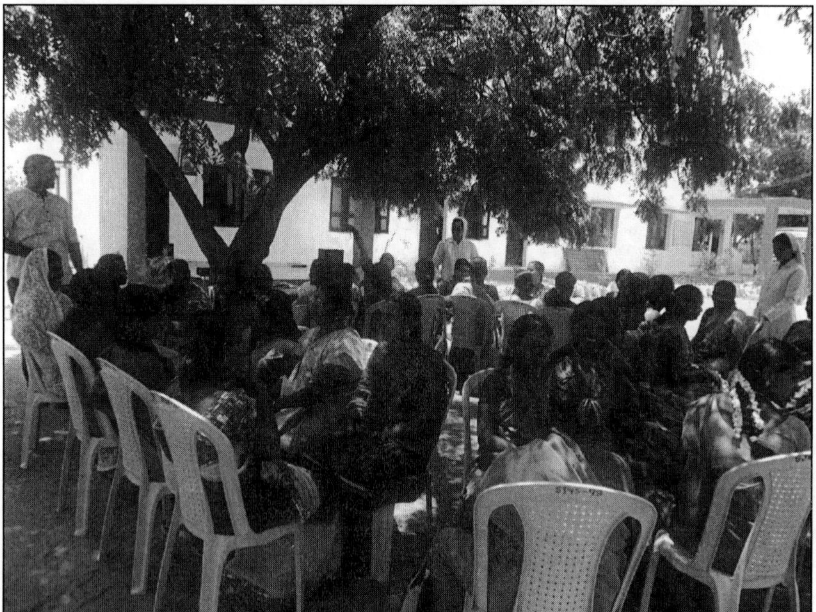

Awareness Programme

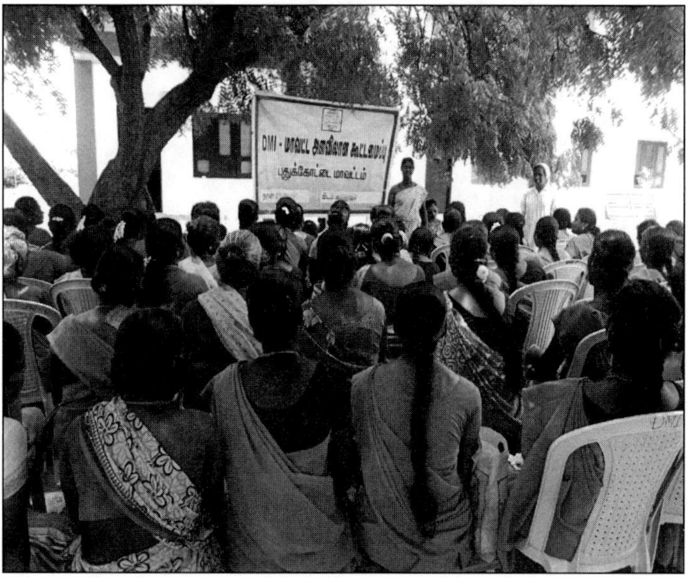

Awareness Programme

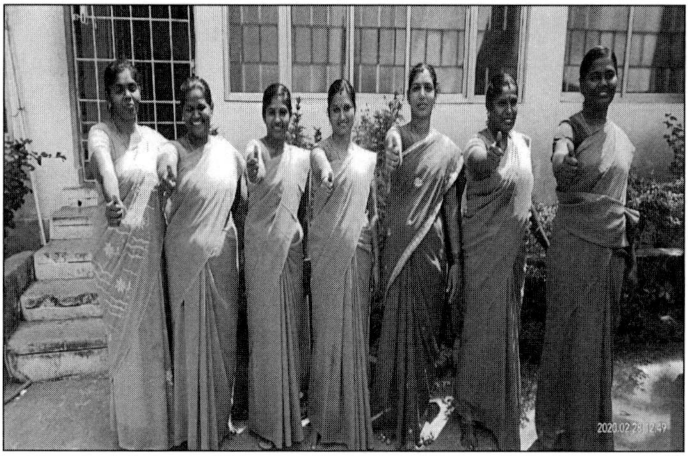

Taking pledge

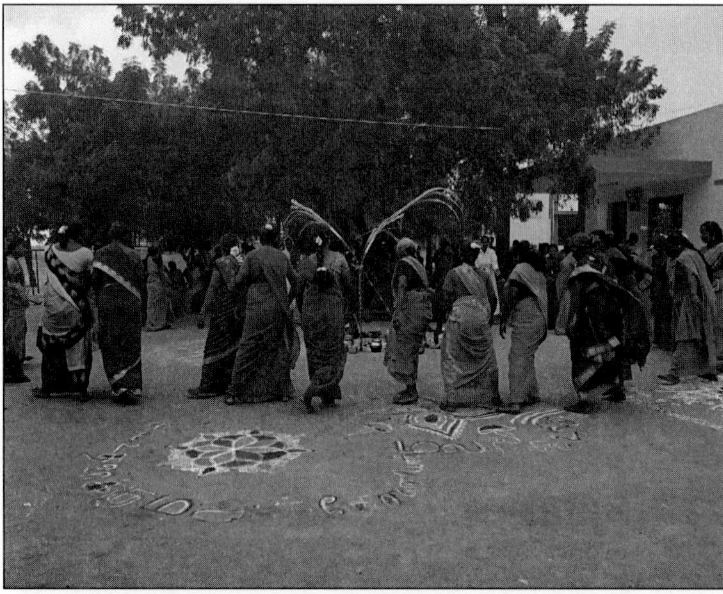

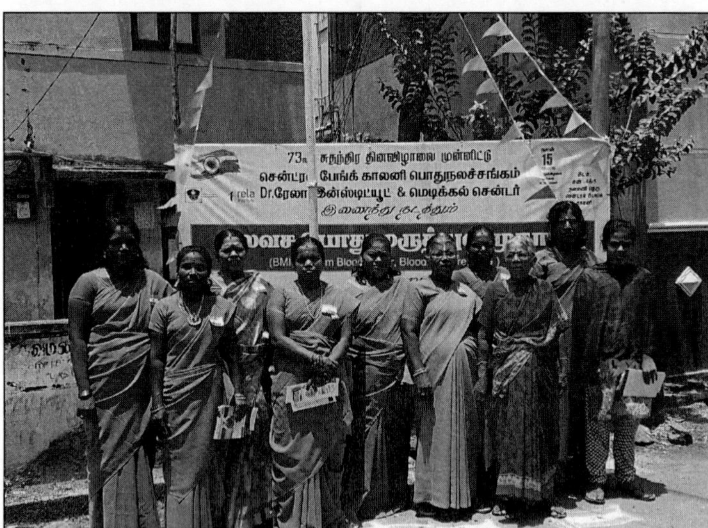
73
சுதந்திர தினவிழாவை முன்னிட்டு
பேங்க் காலனி பொதுநலச்சங்கம்
இன்ஸ்டிட்யூட் & மெடிக்கல் சென்டர்
இணைந்து நடத்தும்
15

Cultural Progamme on Independence Day

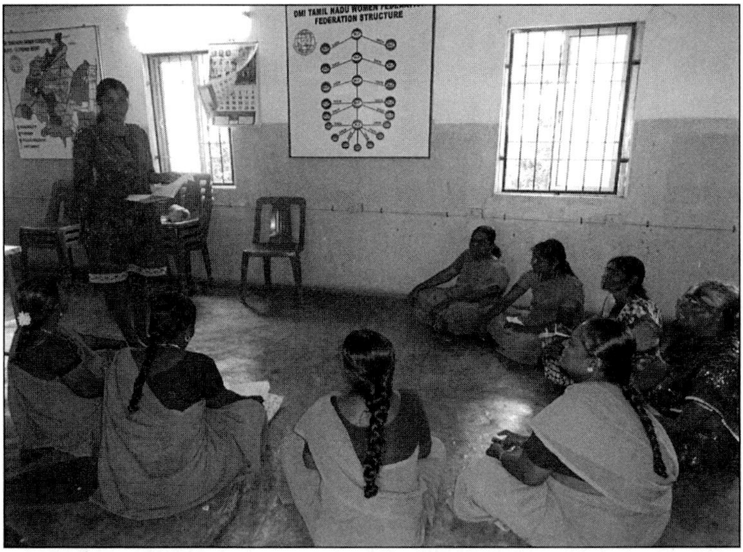

Lecture on HIV/AIDS

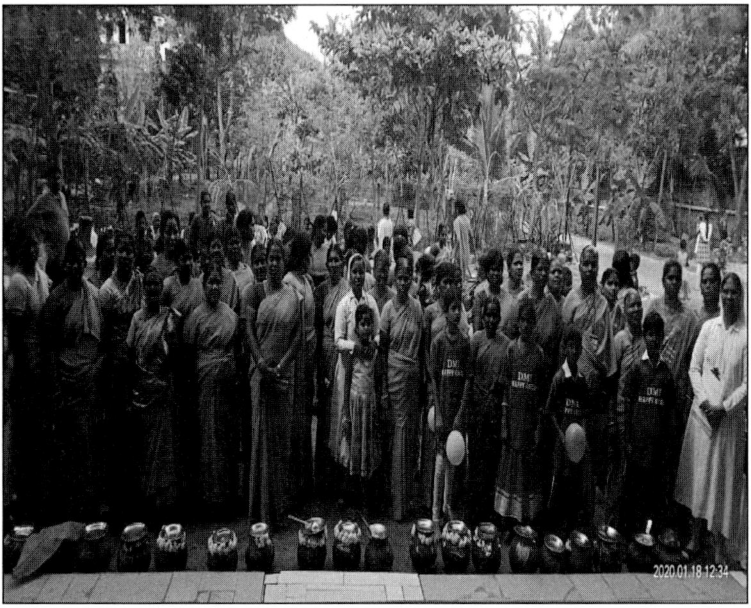

Volunteers with Participants

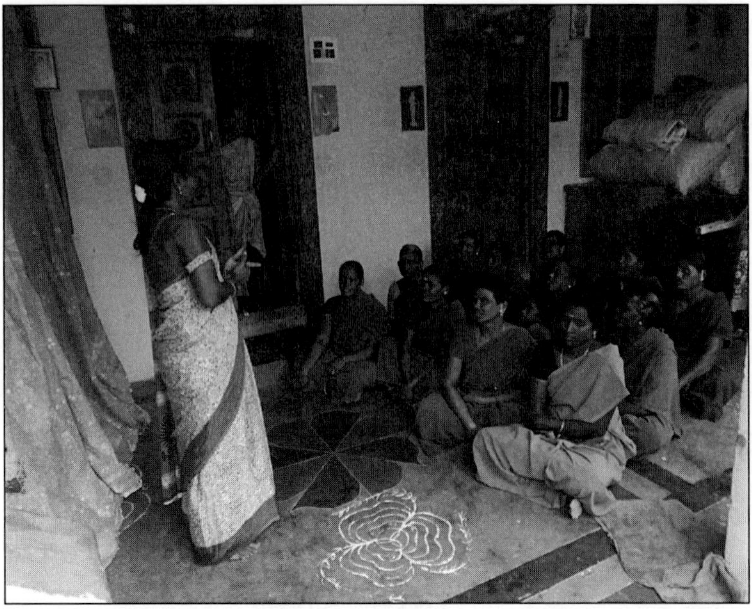

Awareness Lecture

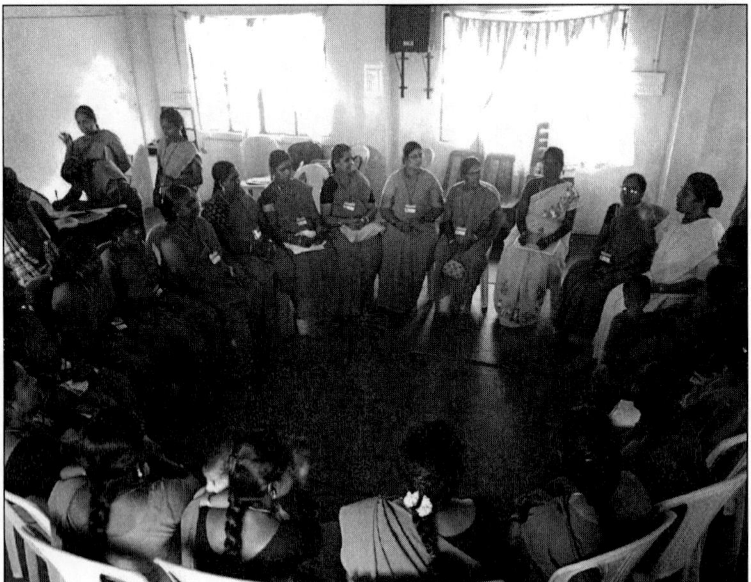

Final Round of sharing and discussion after every programme

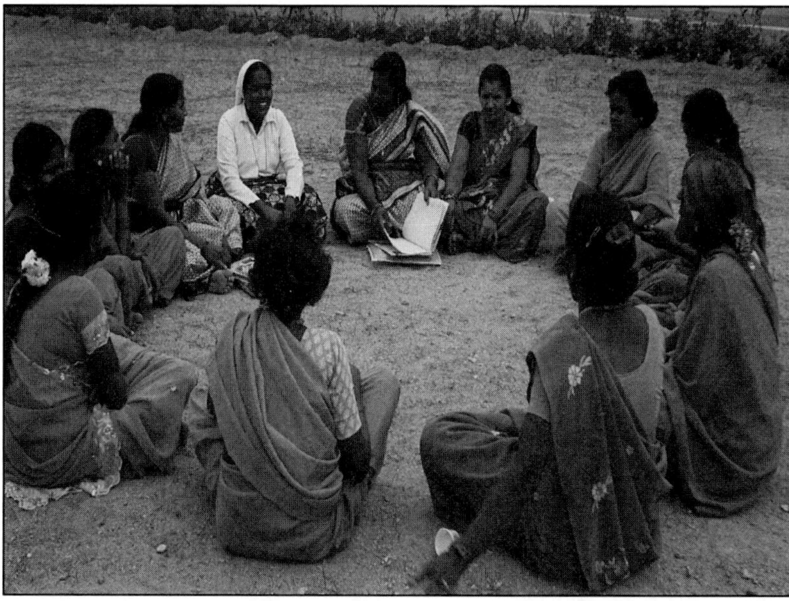

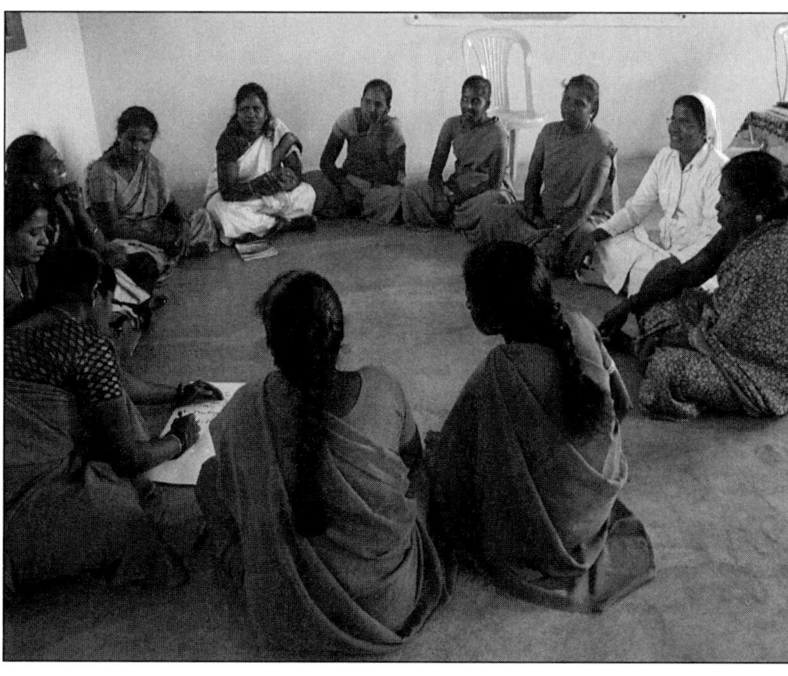

Final Round of sharing and discussion after every programme

Bibliography

Albert. A (1986) Book's Name, *Acquired Immune Deficiency Syndrome,* The Victim and the Press: Studies in Communications, 3, 135 to 158

Altman. D (1986) Book's Name: *AIDS in the Mind of America,* Publisher: New York: Double Day Press.

Atton. C (2000) Book's Name, *Alternative Media.* Publishers: London, Sage.

Bayer. R (1991), Book, *Covering the Plague*, AIDS and the Media. AIDS – Educational and Prevention. 3, 1, 74-86.

Berridge. V. (1994), Book, *AIDS: History and Contemporary History*, The Time of AIDS. Social Analysis, Theory and Method. Publisher: London, Sage.

W.B. Vasantha Kandasamy (2005), Translation by Meena Kandasamy Book: *Fuzzy and Neutrosophic Analysis of Women with HIV/AIDS* with Specific reference to Rural Tamil Nadu.

Arvind Singhal (1999), Book, *The Status of Entertainment* Publisher: Ohio University, U.S.A

Lichtentein (2001), Book, *HIV/AIDS and the Mind* Publisher: Barnes & Nobles.

Davidson Chukwuma Umeh (1997), Book, *Confronting AIDS Epidemic: A Cross-Cultural Perspective on HIV/AIDS Education* Publisher: African World Press, New York.

Gokulsingh (2004), Book, *Soft-Soaping India: The World of Indian Televised Soap Operas.* Publisher: India Book House, New Delhi.

Gabriele Griffin (2001), Book, *Representations of HIV and AIDS,* Visibility Blue/s Publisher: Manchester University Press, England.

Mohan Rao (2004), Book, U*nheard Scream: Reproductive Health and Women's Lives in India*, Publisher: Panaon Institute, India, Zubaan.

You And Aids – The HIV/AIDS Portal for Asia Pacific (Inter-net website)

Elizabeith Manjorie Proude (2006), Book, *HIV/Prevention in General Practice* Publisher: Oxford University Press.

Article: *The History of HIV/AIDS in 20th Anniversay of First AIDS Cases.* U.N. Declaration 2001. New York Press Publications.

Claire Selltiz and others (1962), Book, *Research Methods in Social Sciences* Publisher, American Press.

Ram Ahuja (1992), Book, *Social Problems in India Publisher: Asian Trading Corporation*, New Delhi.

Susan C. Seymour (1997), Book, *Women, Family and child care in India* Publishers: Anandi Press complex, Patna.

The article HIV/AIDS prevention and creating awareness and the role of media by Jyoti singh.boloji.com feb17, 2007.

Indian Prime Minister's speech on the role of media for HIV/AIDS prevention on Jan 06, 2005 http:www. Aids channel.org

Assessing effects of a media campaign on HIV/AIDS prevention in Nigeria; results from the VISION project Joseph Keating, Dominique Meekers, and Alfred Adewuyi BMC Public Health 2006.6.123.

Tamil Nadu State AIDS control society community need assessment programme

Role of communication in HIV prevention Aids free TN.com

Making waves stories of participatory communication for social change. Nalamdana 1993 India.

http://tiruvallur.nic.in/departments/drda.htm

http://www.tn.gov.in/dtp/shg.htm

http://tiruvallur.nic.in/departments/drda.htm

Questionnaire

A COMPARATIVE STUDY ON ROLE OF MEDIA IN CREATING AWARENESS ON HIV/ AIDS AMONG RURAL AND URBAN SELF HELP GROUP MEMBERS WITH PARTICULAR REFERENCE TO KEECHELAM (RURAL) SAIDAPET IN (URBAN)

1. Name
2. Age
3. Gender
4. Education
5. Occupation
6. Income
7. Family Information

No	Relation	Age	Sex	Education	Profession	Inco me	Anyother

AWARENESS ON HIV/AIDS

1. What do you understand by HIV or AIDS?

a) It is a very serious sickness
b) It kills many people
c) I do not know the seriousness
d) I know nothing about it

2. HIV/AIDS is caused by

a) Virus
b) Bacteria
c) Fungus
d) Don't know

3. HIV/ AIDS is a problem of homosexuals

a) Yes
b) No
c) Don't know

4. In your opinion, what is the worst killer disease in our country?

a) Cancer
b) T.B
c) Heart disease
d) HIV/AIDS
e) Any other

5. As for as HIV is concerned, what is its status in India?

a) First
b) Second
c) Third
d) Any other

6. What are the symptoms?

a) Fever
b) Tiredness
c) Loss of weight
d) Not feeling hungry
e) Any other

7. Do you know how long a person will live with AIDS?

a) Approximately 5 years
b) Approximately 10 years
c) Approximately 15 years
d) Do not know

8. I became deeply aware of the problems of HIV/AIDS through

a) TV programs

b) Radio
c) Movies
d) Any other

9. In what way could we use the media in a better way to bring about more awareness?

a) Discussion
b) Open sharing
c) Preventive care Counseling centre
d) Do not know

10. In your knowledge, how does media project the spread of Virus?

a) Sharing of clothes
b) Pregnant mother to child
c) Unsafe sex
d) Infected blood
e) Don't know

11. Does HIV spread from mother to child?

Yes No

12. Media educate that if you take the drug Navarapin, the child will not be affected by HIV/AIDS

Yes No

MEDIA INFORMATION SOURCE

13. What are the different forms of media you have in your house?

a) TV
b) Radio
c) Newspaper
d) Magazine
e) Any other

14. I came to know the most about HIV/AIDS through

a) TV

b) Radio
c) Magazine
d) Newspaper
e) Any other

15. Which is your favorite programme?

a) Serials
b) Advertisements
c) Sports
d) Health related
e) Any other

16. Do you think media should do more to give awareness on aids?

Yes No

17. Do you think media are powerful to bring social awareness in Tamil Nadu on HIV/AIDS?

Yes No

18. Any latest cinema or TV program, you have seen on HIV

Yes No

POSITIVE ATTITUDE TOWARDS HIV/AIDS PATIENT

19. I strongly feel that media can play a significant role to bring out the right attitude on HIV patients.

Yes No

20. I learnt from media that eating with HIV/AIDS patients is not harmful.

Yes No

21. Media taught me that I can exchange my dress and other materials with the HIV/AIDS patients without being affected.

Yes No

22. TV, radio, magazines and newspapers on HIV/AIDS have helped me to change my attitude towards the people affected by HIV/AIDS

Yes No

23. My attitude towards the HIV/AIDS affected patients has changed due to Media information.

Yes No

MEDIA METHODS OF PREVENTION

24. Do you know HIV/AIDS can be prevented through media?

Yes No

25. Have you ever come across any program in TV or Radio on HIV/AIDS prevention method

Yes No

26. How can you prevent getting AIDS?

a) Protected sex
b) Faithful partner
c) Use condom
d) Do not know

27 Has any medium helped you to know about prevention methods?

Yes No

28. Have you heard from the Media the usage of condom?

Yes No

29. Do you think media can help safe blood transfusion to stop spread of HIV/AIDS?

Yes No

30. Do you think media can educate on safe sex to stop spread of HIV/AIDS?

Yes No

Index